THOMSON DELMAR LEARNING'S
CASE STUDY SERIES

Psychiatric Nursing

Betty Kehl Richardson

PhD, RN, CNS-MHP, BC, LPC, LMFT

THOMSON
™
DELMAR LEARNING

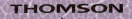

Australia   Canada   Mexico   Singapore   Spain   United Kingdom   United States

THOMSON

DELMAR LEARNING

Thomson Delmar Learning's Case Study Series: Psychiatric Nursing
by Betty Kehl Richardson, PhD, RN, CNS-MHP, BC, LPC, LMFT

**Vice President,
Health Care Business Unit:**
William Brottmiller

Director of Learning Solutions:
Matthew Kane

Acquisitions Editor:
Maureen Rosener

Product Manager:
Elizabeth Howe

Editorial Assistant:
Chelsey Iaquinta

Marketing Director:
Jennifer McAvey

Marketing Manager:
Michele McTighe

Marketing Coordinator:
Danielle Pacella

Production Director:
Carolyn Miller

Content Project Manager:
Jessica McNavich

Library of Congress Cataloging-in-Publication Data

Richardson, Betty Kehl.
   Psychiatric nursing/Betty Kehl
   Richardson.
     p. ; cm. —
   (Thomson Delmar Learning's case study series)
   Includes bibliographical references and index.
   ISBN 1-4018-3847-2 (pbk. : alk. paper)
  1. Psychiatric nursing—Case studies.
 I. Title. II. Series.
   [DNLM: 1. Psychiatric Nursing—methods—Case Reports.
 2. Psychiatric Nursing—methods—Problems and Exercises. 3. Mental Disorders—nursing—Case Reports.
 4. Mental Disorders—nursing—Problems and Exercises. WY 160 R521p 2007]

RC440.R53 2007
616.89'0231—dc22
                       2006015981

Notice to the Reader

Contents

Reviewers

Ann K. Beckett, PhD, RN
Assistant Professor
Oregon Health and Science University School of Nursing
Portland, Oregon

Jane E. Bostick, PhD, APRN, BC
Assistant Professor of Clinical Nursing
University of Missouri–Columbia
Sinclair School of Nursing
Columbia, Missouri

Kimberly M. Gregg, MS APRN, BC
Adult Mental Health Clinical Nurse Specialist
Altru Health Systems
Instructor
University of North Dakota
Grand Forks, North Dakota

Bethany Phoenix, RN, PhD, CNS
Associate Clinical Professor
Coordinator, Graduate Program in Psychiatric/Mental
Health Nursing
University of California, San Francisco
San Francisco, California

Charlotte R. Price, EdD, RN
Professor and Chair
Augusta State University Department of Nursing
Augusta, Georgia

Linda Stafford, PhD, RN, CS
Division Head, Psychiatric Mental Health Nursing
The University of Texas Health Science Center at Houston
School of Nursing
Houston, Texas

Preface

Thomson Delmar Learning's Case Studies Series was created to encourage nurses to bridge the gap between content knowledge and clinical application. The products within the series represent the most innovative and comprehensive approach to nursing case studies ever developed. Each title has been authored by experienced nurse educators and clinicians who understand the complexity of nursing practice as well as the challenges of teaching and learning. All of the cases are based on real-life clinical scenarios and demand thought and "action" from the nurse. Each case brings the user into the clinical setting, and invites him or her to utilize the nursing process while considering all of the variables that influence the client's condition and the care to be provided. Each case also represents a unique set of variables, to offer a breadth of learning experiences and to capture the reality of nursing practice. To gauge the progression of a user's knowledge and critical thinking ability, the cases have been categorized by difficulty level. Every section begins with basic cases and proceeds to more advanced scenarios, thereby presenting opportunities for learning and practice for both students and professionals.

All of the cases have been expert reviewed to ensure that as many variables as possible are represented in a truly realistic manner and that each case reflects consistency with realities of modern nursing practice.

Praise for Delmar Learning's Case Study Series

"These cases show diversity and richness of content and should stimulate lively discussions with students."

—LINDA STAFFORD, PhD, RN
Division Head, Psychiatric Mental Health Nursing, School of Nursing, The University of Texas Health Science Center at Houston

"The use of case studies is pedagogically sound and very appealing to students and instructors. I think that some instructors avoid them because of the challenge of case development. You have provided the material for them."

—NANCY L. OLDENBURG, RN, MS, CPNP
Clinical Instructor, Northern Illinois University

"[The author] has done an excellent job of assisting students to engage in critical thinking. I am very impressed with the cases, questions, and content. I rarely ask that students buy more than one . . . book . . . but, in this instance, I can't wait until this book is published."

—DEBORAH J. PERSELL, MSN, RN, CPNP
Assistant Professor, Arkansas State University

"[The case studies] are very current and prepare students for the twenty-first-century mental health arena."

—CHARLOTTE R. PRICE, EdD, RN
Professor and Chair, Augusta State University
Department of Nursing

"One thing I always tell my students is that they will encounter mental health issues in all the various areas of nursing that they practice. Often they don't grasp this concept. . . . Many mental health nursing books focus on mental health settings and miss the other settings. I appreciate the fact that different settings were used in this reading . . . inpatient and outpatient, as well as med-surg, plastic surgery, etc."

—KIMBERLY M. GREGG, MS APRN, BC
Adult Mental Health Clinical Nurse Specialist,
Altru Health Systems, Instructor, University of
North Dakota

"This is a groundbreaking book. . . . This book should be a required text for all undergraduate and graduate nursing programs and should be well-received by faculty."

—JANE H. BARNSTEINER, PhD, RN, FAAN
Professor of Pediatric Nursing, University of
Pennsylvania School of Nursing

How to Use this Book

Every case begins with a table of variables that are encountered in practice, and that must be understood by the nurse in order to provide appropriate care to the client. Categories of variables include age, gender, setting, ethnicity, cultural considerations, preexisting conditions, coexisting conditions, communication considerations, disability considerations, socioeconomic considerations, spiritual considerations, pharmacological considerations, psychosocial considerations, legal considerations, ethical considerations, alternative therapy, prioritization considerations, and delegation considerations. If a case involves a variable that is considered to have a significant impact on care, the specific variable is included in the table. This allows the user an "at a glance" view of the issues that will need to be considered to provide care to the client in the scenario. The table of variables is followed by a presentation of the case, including the history of the client, current condition, clinical setting, and professionals involved. A series of questions follows each case that ask the user to consider how she would handle the issues presented within the scenario. Suggested answers and rationales are provided for remediation and discussion.

Organization

Cases are grouped according to psychiatric disorder. Within each part, cases are organized by difficulty level from easy, to moderate, to difficult. This classification is somewhat subjective, but they are based upon a developed standard. In general, difficulty level has been determined by the number of variables that impact the case and the complexity of the client's condition. Colored tabs are used to allow the user to distinguish the difficulty levels more easily. A comprehensive table of variables is also provided for reference, to allow the user to quickly select cases containing a particular variable of care.

The cases are fictitious; however, they are based on actual problems and/or situations the nurse will encounter. Any resemblance to actual cases or individuals is coincidental.

Acknowledgments

For the invitation to write this book, the author wishes to express her appreciation to Erin Silk and Matt Kane of Thomson Delmar Publishers. A number of product managers and staff were involved over time, and the author thanks them for their help. The author is most indebted to Elizabeth (Libby) Howe, the final product manager, who provided guidance, feedback, ideas, and encouragement to keep the project alive and get the book into print. Another special thanks goes to Nora Armbruster, who managed the final production stage and made it possible to meet the print deadline. The author wants to especially thank the reviewers and copy editors of this book, for their time, expertise, critical comments, and suggestions, which resulted in changes to make the book much better.

A number of colleagues at Austin Community College, Austin, Texas; Austin State Hospital; and Seton Shoal Creek Psychiatric Hospital, as well as other psychiatric and medical facilities, were consulted about selected aspects of the cases to verify accuracy and currency. The author recognizes and appreciates the important contributions of these colleagues: Sally Samford, Marita Peppard, Donna Edwards, Kris Benton, Kitty Viek, Jane Luetchens, and many others.

Teachers and school nurses were consulted, as were parents of children with special issues. The author wishes to recognize their important contributions, especially Edna Nation, who teaches high school students in Liberty Hill, Texas, for her dedication to helping all students—including those with medical and mental health problems—achieve their maximum potential and for sharing her ideas with the author.

The author thanks her family and friends for their patience and understanding during the long months of research and writing. This project could not have been finished without their encouragement and cooperation.

Dedication

This book is dedicated to my son Mark, who has battled cancer throughout most of the time this book was in progress. Sharing with me some of his innermost thoughts, fears, and struggles has reinforced for me that what student nurses, family, and others see on the surface in a brief interaction with a client can be a very different picture than what is going on inside the client. Compassion, empathy, and therapeutic communication do help us understand that inner person. I am indebted to Mark for all he has taught me.

Additionally, this book is dedicated to all the good nurses in various fields of nursing, not just psychiatric mental health nursing, who apply psychiatric techniques and principles when working with clients who have mental health diagnoses and/or issues.

Note from the Author

These case studies were designed to help nursing students at all levels to not only fine tune their critical thinking skills and their therapeutic communication skills, but to develop a deeper understanding of, and empathy for, clients who have what we currently refer to as psychiatric problems. The mind and body are inseparable, so physical health problems are interwoven with mental health problems within the cases. The student nurse, and anyone else who reads these case studies, is encouraged to ask themselves: "What is the most therapeutic approach or response to this client in this situation?" as they answer the questions within the cases.

About the Author

Dr. Richardson began a nursing career in 1959 as a new diploma graduate. She worked five years in obstetrical nursing at Memorial Medical Center, Springfield, Illinois; much of this time she worked in the labor rooms and applied nearly everything she learned in psychiatric nursing to emotionally support laboring women, new mothers, and grieving parents who lost babies. She next worked as an office nurse for Dr. Tom Masters, a general internist who specialized in Diabetes. The following several years she worked for the Illinois Department of Mental Health Mental Retardation, working on an outpatient team serving three rural counties. The team followed the blurred role concept in which every member did intake evaluations and did counseling with people having the full range of diagnoses and issues possible in mental health work. This work stimulated a return to school for a bachelor's in nursing and a master's in administration from the University of Illinois at Springfield, a master's degrees in adult nursing from the Medical College of Georgia, and a PhD in psychiatric mental health nursing from the University of Texas at Austin, Texas. Her dissertation was "The Psychiatric Inpatient's Perception of the Seclusion Room Experience." She published the results of this study in *Nursing Research.* Dr. Richardson has taught in an RN to BSN program, two ADN programs, and a licensed vocational nursing program. She received the NISOD teaching award for teaching excellence from the University of Texas.

Throughout the years, volunteer work has been a passion. Dr. Richardson made fifteen trips to Honduras and Nicaragua with MEDICO, a nonprofit organization taking medical, eye, and dental care to remote areas that are medically underserved. She co-led trips to the Moskito Coast of Nicaragua and Honduras and volunteered for several months in a program to take boys off the streets of LaCeiba, Honduras. Additional volunteer work has been with the homeless in Austin, Texas.

Dr. Richardson is also a licensed professional counselor and a licensed marriage and family therapist and has done therapy for over thirty years (full time and part time). She has worked as a therapist in a residential program for children and adolescents and as a service administrator and therapist on a child/adolescent unit in a private psychiatric hospital. She led weekend groups in a private psychiatric hospital for many years while teaching full time. She was Director of Nursing of Austin State Hospital, Austin, Texas, for six years. Over the years, Dr. Richardson has had training with a number of the great theorists such as Bettleheim, Azrin, Frankl, Ellis, and others. She has had training in a variety of therapies from Psychoanalytic Theory to Play Therapy to Brief Psychotherapy. She is a board-certified clinical specialist in child adolescent psychiatric nursing (certified by the American Nurses Association). She continues in her private practice, works part time in a drug study clinic, freelances for publishers, and has written a monthly column for parents in the newsmagazine *Austin Parent* since 1992. Dr. Richardson has lived in Austin, Texas, for over twenty-five years, and she can be contacted there by e-mail at bkrich@sbcglobal.net.

Comprehensive Table of Variables

Case Study	Gender	Age	Setting	Ethnicity	Culture	Preexisting Conditions	Coexisting Conditions	Communication	Disability	Socioeconomic Status	Spirituality	Pharmacologic	Psychosocial	Legal	Ethical	Alternative Therapy	Prioritization	Delegation
Part One: The Client Experiencing Schizophrenia and Other Psychotic Disorders																		
1	M	23	Hospital	White American						X		X	X	X	X		X	
2	M	68	Home	White American		X				X		X	X	X				
Part Two: The Client Experiencing Anxiety																		
1	M	14	School nurse	Turkish American	X							X		X	X			
2	F	25	Clinic	White American	X				X	X	X	X		X	X	X		
Part Three: The Client Experiencing Depression or Mania																		
1	M	12	Center	White American	X					X			X	X	X	X		
2	F	22	Clinic	White American			X				X							
Part Four: The Client Who Abuses Chemical Substances																		
1	M	43	Center	White American	X					X	X	X	X	X	X	X		
2	M	25	Resid. facility	Black American	X	X	X			X	X		X	X	X	X		
3	F	20	Resid. facility	White American		X				X			X	X				
Part Five: The Client with a Personality Disorder																		
1	F	28	Hospital	White American									X				X	
2	M	20	City jail	White American	X		X			X		X	X	X	X	X	X	
3	M	37	Hospital	Mexican American			X			X			X	X	X	X		

Part Six: The Client Experiencing a Somatoform, Factitious, or Dissociative Disorder

	Sex	Age	Setting	Ethnicity												
1	M	52	Outpatient	White American	X		X		X	X	X	X	X		X	
2	F	24	Office	White American			X		X	X	X	X			
3	F	28	Hospital	White American	X				X	X	X	X	X	X	X

Part Seven: The Client with Disorders of Self-Regulation

	Sex	Age	Setting	Ethnicity												
1	M	30	Clinic	White American	X					X	X				
2	F	14	School nurse	Mexican American	X				X		X				

Part Eight: Special Populations: The Child, Adolescent, or Elderly Client

	Sex	Age	Setting	Ethnicity												
1	F	17	Ob-gyn office	Black American	X					X			X		
2	M	10	Camp	White American	X	X	X	X	X	X	X	X		X	
3	M	75	Retirement	Black American community	X	X	X	X	X	X	X	X			

Part Nine: Survivors of Violence or Abuse

	Sex	Age	Setting	Ethnicity												
1	F	23	Inpatient	White American	X	X	X		X	X	X	X	X	X	

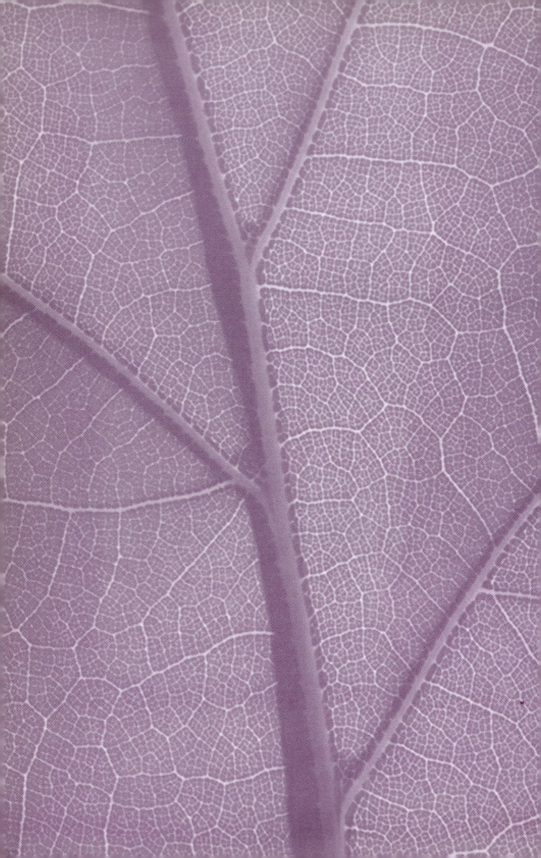

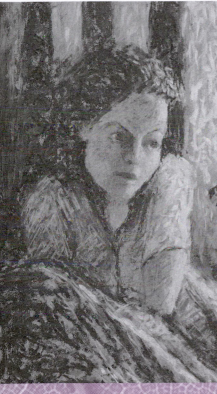

PART ONE

The Client Experiencing Schizophrenia and Other Psychotic Disorders

CASE STUDY 1

Charles

GENDER

M

AGE

23

SETTING

- Hospital

ETHNICITY

- White American

CULTURAL CONSIDERATIONS

PREEXISTING CONDITIONS

COEXISTING CONDITIONS

COMMUNICATION

DISABILITY

SOCIOECONOMIC

- Middle class

SPIRITUAL/RELIGIOUS

PHARMACOLOGIC

- Haloperidol (Haldol)

PSYCHOSOCIAL

- Single-parent family

LEGAL

- Confidentiality

ETHICAL

- Social vs. therapeutic relationship

ALTERNATIVE THERAPY

PRIORITIZATION

- Preventing harm to self or others while establishing a trusting relationship

DELEGATION

MODERATE

SCHIZOPHRENIA AND OTHER PSYCHOTIC DISORDERS

Level of difficulty: Moderate

Overview: This case requires the ability to process and resolve issues associated with the admission and care of a client who demonstrates aggressive behavior, delusions, and hallucinations.

3

Client Profile

Charles is a 23-year-old male graduate student who comes from a single-parent, middle-class family; his father abandoned the family when Charles was a baby. He attends school on scholarship, and his mother works two jobs to help support him. Although Charles has a roommate, they interact infrequently. One day, Charles pins his roommate to the wall and threatens him with a knife while mumbling something about people trying to control his brain through radio waves. Charles accuses the roommate (and others) of trying to poison him. The campus police respond to calls for help.

Case Study

The campus police officer brings Charles to the psychiatric unit of a local hospital. Charles moves to the corner of the room and sits by himself, but remains within eyesight of the police officer and staff. The nurse notices that Charles' lips move occasionally and his head turns as if to hear someone speaking. She also notes that Charles is tall and thin. His appearance is unkempt, with an unshaven face and soiled, wrinkled clothing. He does not make eye contact. Charles seems frightened, yet his manner and history suggest that he poses a threat to others.

The nurse introduces herself to Charles and tells him that he is in a safe place. She speaks softly and slowly, and she chooses her words with care. Then she takes Charles to an office to interview him. She is alone with him, but leaves the office door open. A mental health worker stands outside the door. Charles refuses to sign any information release forms during the admissions process.

Later, the nurse calls medical records for Charles' records from an admission one year ago. The record reveals a diagnosis of Schizophrenia, Paranoid Type and that Charles was discharged on haloperidol (Haldol) and referred to the college health center psychiatrist. Charles tells the nurse he has not been taking the haloperidol. The nurse calls the admitting psychiatrist for orders. The psychiatrist debates whether to put Charles back on haloperidol or prescribe a newer atypical antipsychotic/neuroleptic. The nurse then receives a call from Charles' mother. She questions whether Charles is there and asks to speak to him. When the nurse tries to tell Charles that his mother has called, Charles asks whether she is married, where she lives, and if he may see her after he is discharged.

Questions

1. What is the significance of Charles' appearance and behavior?

2. Which signs and symptoms match the criteria for Schizophrenia?

3. What are the positive and negative signs and symptoms of Schizophrenia? Which ones does Charles manifest?

4. Which subtype of Schizophrenia do Charles' signs and symptoms suggest?

5. What provisional nursing diagnoses could be made based on the limited data available? Which one would rank as the top priority?

6. With what basic issues is the nurse dealing?

7. What does the nurse do to protect herself from Charles? What else could she do?

8. How should the nurse deal with the mother's inquiry and request? Why?

9. What would be the most therapeutic response the nurse could offer Charles when he talks about his delusions or admits to hearing voices or other hallucinations?

10. If you were Charles' nurse, what response would you give to questions about your marital status and dating availability? How would you feel if you were asked these questions?

11. What is Charles' developmental stage? What are the tasks of that stage (use Erickson's or Havinghurst's theories of developmental stages)?

12. If you were the nurse, how would you respond to Charles' admission that he had stopped taking haloperidol? Discuss haloperidol and older neuroleptics as well as newer atypical neuroleptics.

13. In addition to medication, what other treatments might be used with Charles and other clients with Schizophrenia?

Questions and Suggested Answers

1. What is the significance of Charles' appearance and behavior? Charles' appearance suggests that he is not attending to personal hygiene (shaving or changing his clothes). He is thin and likely not consuming enough calories; he might be dehydrated as well. He says he believes he is being poisoned. As the nurse develops rapport with the client, she might offer him unopened cartons of milk, juice, and/or bottled water or get him to eat a microwavable dinner presented in an unopened box ready for microwaving.

Pinning a roommate to the wall with a knife, fearing that others will harm him, and appearing to respond to voices indicate that Charles poses a danger to others. He might feel that he must hurt others before they hurt him, or he might respond affirmatively to voices commanding him to hurt others.

2. Which signs and symptoms match the criteria for Schizophrenia? To meet the requirements for a diagnosis for Schizophrenia, a person must exhibit two or more of five characteristic symptoms, and each symptom

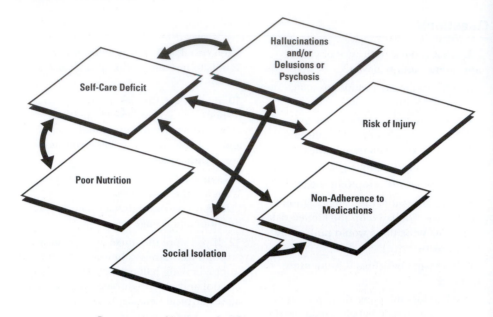

Concept map of issues and problems associated with schizophrenia.

must have been present for a significant amount of time during a month. The five symptoms are delusions, hallucinations, disorganized speech, grossly disorganized or catatonic behavior, and negative symptoms (e.g., affective flattening, alogia, or avolition). Under special circumstances, the presence of delusions or hallucinations is enough. There must be a disturbance in one or more major areas of functioning for a significant portion of time, the continuous signs of the disturbance must persist for at least six months, and other possible causes of these symptoms must be ruled out (APA, 2000).

3. What are the positive and negative signs and symptoms of Schizophrenia? Which ones does Charles manifest? Positive symptoms of schizophrenia represent an excess or distortion of normal functions. Positive symptoms include delusions, hallucinations, disorganized speech, and disorganized or catatonic behavior. Negative symptoms include a diminution or loss of normal functions as well as affective flattening, alogia (poverty of speech), and avolition (lack of motivation). Relative to positive signs, Charles is experiencing persecutory delusions and might be hallucinating. As for negative signs, Charles manifests avolition by failing to bathe and complete other hygiene chores.

4. Which subtype of Schizophrenia do Charles' signs and symptoms suggest? Paranoid-Type Schizophrenia is suggested. In Paranoid-Type

Schizophrenia, the client is preoccupied with one or more delusions typically persecutory or grandiose or both, or frequent auditory hallucinations. Disorganized speech, disorganized or catatonic behavior, or flat or inappropriate affect is not present. The client is preoccupied with thoughts of being harmed by others.

5. What provisional nursing diagnoses could be made based on the limited data available? Which one would rank as the top priority? The provisional nursing diagnoses include risk for other-directed violence; imbalanced nutrition: less-than-body requirements; bathing/hygiene self-care deficit; dressing/grooming self-care deficit; disturbed thought processes; disturbed sensory perceptions; social isolation; and medication noncompliance. The top priority would be risk for other-directed violence. Depending on the data, other potential diagnoses arising from the assessment findings include ineffective role performance and knowledge deficit (NANDA, 2005), among others.

6. With what basic issues is the nurse dealing? The basic issues include safety, trust, confidentiality, physiologic needs (nutrition and fluids), companionship needs, and a sense of belonging. The nurse must protect the client from harming others and stay safe herself. At the same time, the nurse must increase the client's interactions with others in a safe and therapeutic manner. McDonald and Badger (2002,42) state that "positive social relationships, or positive social function have been found to decrease hospitalizations and shorten lengths of stay for persons with schizophrenia."

7. What does the nurse do to protect herself from Charles? What else could she do? The nurse begins by introducing herself. She speaks softly and slowly, as clients with a diagnosis of Schizophrenia often are sensitive to noise, light, and other forms of sensory stimulation. In addition, the nurse assures the client that he is in a safe place and does not need to fight to protect himself. The nurse keeps the door open during the client interview and places a mental health worker outside the door to help if needed.

Additional precautions the nurse could take include sitting between the client and the door and staying alert for behavioral clues that the client is escalating (e.g., foot tapping, hypervigilance, and verbal clues such as a raised voice and threat issuance).

The nurse needs to keep at least an arm's length between the client and herself. If the nurse must be closer to do a procedure, the nurse should explain the procedure first and then ask permission to approach the client. The nurse can help de-escalate the client's mood by noting evident emotions, encouraging the client to describe how he feels, and listening to the client.

The nurse must be trained in acceptable, effective methods for management of aggressive behavior that comply with hospital policies and procedures and state regulations.

8. How should the nurse deal with the mother's inquiry and request? Why? The client's refusal to sign a release of information form makes it impossible for the nurse to tell the mother—or anyone else—that Charles is in the hospital. The nurse could respond by telling the mother that this information is not available. Most mental health care facilities support a nurse telling family members that they can leave a telephone number in case their loved one is in the hospital or later admitted.

9. What would be the most therapeutic response the nurse could offer Charles when he talks about his delusions or admits to hearing voices or other hallucinations? *Delusions* are fixed, false beliefs; thus, no argument or logic will change the client's delusions. Therefore, it is best to avoid asking the client to tell you more about them. With medication, a therapeutic environment, rest, and other changes, the delusions will stop. *Hallucinations* are false perceptions involving any of the senses; auditory hallucinations (hearing voices) are the most common form. The best nursing approach is to advise clients that you understand that they hear, see, smell, or feel hallucinations, but that you do not. Because clients seem to hallucinate more when isolated, interventions often seek to reduce isolation and keep clients busy.

10. If you were Charles' nurse, what response would you give to questions about your marital status and dating availability? How would you feel if you were asked these questions? It is neither necessary nor helpful for the client to focus on the nurse's marital status or other personal information, even though the client might be able to overhear clues or make accurate guesses. Acceptable therapeutic responses include refocusing or redirecting the client, saying something like, "Let's focus on you. You were saying earlier____." Some nurses have difficulty asking clients for information without giving clients equivalent information about themselves in exchange. Such nurses can benefit from a review of therapeutic versus social communication.

Nurses admit to a variety of feelings when clients exhibit interest in a personal relationship with the nurse. Feelings range from being flattered and excited to being shocked and angry. While any feeling that the nurse might have is understandable, the range of acceptable responses is limited. It is unprofessional for the nurse to engage in a personal relationship with a client. The nurse can gently remind the client of their nurse–client relationship and let the client know what the nurse can do to help them stay within the professional boundaries.

11. What is Charles' developmental stage? What are the tasks of that stage (use Erickson's or Havinghurst's theories of developmental stages)? According to Erickson (Frisch and Frisch, 2006, 42), a person age 18 to 25 is in the stage of intimacy versus isolation. The task of this stage is to find a life mate. Havinghurst (Ramont and Niedringhaus, 2004, 606) identifies the developmental tasks of early adulthood as selecting a partner, learning to live with a partner, starting a family, and managing a home. Looking at this client's developmental tasks, the nurse can understand that his interest in a personal relationship is normal behavior for this stage in life, even though the nurse cannot engage in such a relationship and must set limits as well as guide interactions with the client in a therapeutic and professional manner.

12. If you were the nurse, how would you respond to Charles' admission that he had stopped taking haloperidol? Discuss haloperidol and older neuroleptics as well as newer atypical neuroleptics. In order to develop a plan to increase medication compliance, the nurse must determine why Charles stopped taking his medication. The nurse could say something such as, "Tell me about what was going on that caused you to stop the medication." The reasons for noncompliance with medication regimens vary, but could include a perceived lack of therapeutic response, side effects, financial concerns about the cost of medication, and difficulties accessing the system to get prescriptions (Beebe, 2002).

Haloperidol is one of the older antipsychotics in use today. It helps improve behavior patterns and reduce agitation, hostility, psychosis, and delusions. It comes as an oral concentrate, a tablet, and a long-acting decanoate, which must be given deep intramuscularly (IM) every three to four weeks. Haloperidol is helpful in clients who are noncompliant in taking a daily pill (Spratto and Woods, 2006). It can cause significant extrapyramidal effects, anticholinergic effects (e.g., dry mouth and constipation), and orthostatic hypotension. Frisch and Frisch (2006) indicate that typical neuroleptics such as haloperidol and chlorpromazine (Thorazine) act similarly on symptoms of Schizophrenia, with greater effect on positive symptoms and less effect on negative symptoms, which tends to leave clients socially incapacitated. Unlike older neuroleptics, newer neuroleptics, often called atypical neuroleptics, are more effective in reducing negative symptoms and do not seem to cause movement disorders at usual doses. Atypical neuroleptics include clozapine (Clozaril), Olanzapine (Zyprexia), reserpine (Risperidol), quetiapine (Seroquel), ziprasidone (Geodon), and aripiprazole (Abilify). These medications are not without side effects or problems, however. Clozapine requires careful monitoring of white blood cell counts as it can cause severe agranulocytosis, which could be fatal. Ziprasidone and Olanzapine have a risk for a prolonged QT/QTc interval, which has been associated with a potentially fatal type of arrhythmia: torsade de points (Spratto and Woods, 2006). The newer antipsychotic medications might work better for some clients, while others will do well on older antipsychotics. Newer antipsychotic medications are much more expensive.

Schizophrenia affects all communities worldwide but there might "be genetically determined pharmacodynamic differences between ethnic groups" (Emsely, 2004, 22). Black Americans are more likely to get higher doses of antipsychotics, while white Americans are more likely to get depot injections. Asian clients get lower doses than white Americans due to findings of higher plasma concentrations of antipsychotics in this group (Emsley, 2004).

13. In addition to medication, what other treatments might be used with Charles and other clients with Schizophrenia? Two main approaches prevail in the treatment of Schizophrenia: the psychosocial approach and the pharmacologic approach. Nurses exercise a collaborative role in each, assisting other professionals in providing psychosocial therapies and in monitoring pharmacologic treatment (Frisch and Frisch, 2006). Psychosocial approaches rely on a variety of tools, including teaching the client stress management skills, leisure skills, and assertiveness, and educating the client about his or her mental illness and its treatment. Nurses also play important roles in supporting the client's family

References

American Psychiatric Association (APA). (2000). *Diagnostic and Statistical Manual of Mental Disorders, 4th ed.* Text Revision. Washington, DC: APA.

Beebe, L. H. (2002). "Problems in Community Living Identified by People with Schizophrenia." *Journal of Psychosocial Nursing* 40(2): 38–45.

Emsley, R. (2004). "Ethnicity and Treatment Response in Schizophrenia." *Psychiatric Times* 21(8): 21–23.

Frisch, N. C. and L. E. Frisch. (2006). *Psychiatric Mental Health Nursing, 3d ed.* Albany, NY: Thomson Delmar Learning.

McDonald, J. and T. A. Badger. (2002). "Social Function of Persons with Schizophrenia." *Journal of Psychosocial Nursing* 40(6): 42–44.

North American Nursing Diagnosis Association (NANDA). (2005). *Nursing Diagnoses: Definitions and Classification 2005–2006.* Philadelphia: NANDA.

Ramont, R. P. and D. M. Niedringhaus. (2003). *Fundamental Nursing Care.* Upper Saddle River, N. J.: Pearson Prentice Hall.

Spratto, G. R. and A. L. Woods. (2006). *PDR Nurse's Drug Handbook.* Clifton Park, NY: Thomson Delmar Learning.

Ben

GENDER

   M

AGE

   68

SETTING

- Home visit by visiting nurse

ETHNICITY

- White American

CULTURAL CONSIDERATIONS

- Grew up in a rural, hill-country counterculture. Lived in a counterculture commune
  in the 1960s and now once again lives
  in the counterculture of his youth. Is a
  member of motorcycle club with its own
  culture

PREEXISTING CONDITIONS

- Paranoia of undetermined origin or cause

COEXISTING CONDITIONS

COMMUNICATION

DISABILITY

SOCIOECONOMIC

- Lower middle income; collects Social
  Security

SPIRITUAL/RELIGIOUS

PHARMACOLOGIC

- Haloperidol (Haldol) decanoate
- Prochlorperazine (Compazine)

PSYCHOSOCIAL

- Paranoia interferes with socialization in
  general and intimacy with wife

LEGAL

- Risk of lawsuit if client develops
  Neuroleptic Malignant Syndrome (NMS)

ETHICAL

ALTERNATIVE THERAPY

PRIORITIZATION

DELEGATION

MODERATE

SCHIZOPHRENIA AND OTHER PSYCHOTIC DISORDERS

Level of difficulty: Moderate

Overview: Requires knowledge of the symptoms of NMS, the ability to recognize them in
clients, and the use of critical thinking to determine an appropriate course of action when
these symptoms present.

Client Profile

Ben is a 68-year-old male who grew up in the hill country, the child of anti-establishment, counterculture parents. Ben took a few college classes with no particular goals and lived in a commune in the 1960s. When his parents died, he married his girlfriend, and they moved into his deceased parents' home. He and his wife currently receive Social Security income. Ben admits to experimenting with illegal drugs in the past, but claims he is clean now. While suffering from paranoia for several years, his condition began to deteriorate recently, and he is now experiencing hallucinations. The exact cause of his paranoia is unknown because Ben refuses to accept psychiatric treatment. Recently, Ben has isolated himself from his motorcycle club. He thinks his wife, Marie, is trying to poison him; he also believes she is hiding money and secretly planning to leave him. Marie and some friends finally convince Ben to see a psychiatrist by recommending one who shares Ben's interest in motorcycles.

After doing a complete physical and evaluation, the psychiatrist prescribes haloperidol (Haldol) decanoate, a long-lasting depot narcoleptic, prompted by Ben's poor history of complying with medication regimens. The psychiatrist tells Ben a visiting nurse will come to his home monthly to administer the injection.

Case Study

The visiting nurse plans to visit Ben at his home twenty-one days after his first depot injection to administer his next dose of haloperidol decanoate. When the nurse calls to verify the appointment, Marie relates that Ben is not well. When the nurse arrives at the home, he takes Ben's vital signs. His findings are

Temperature (oral): 103° F
Pulse: 136
Respirations: 28
Blood pressure: 148/96

Ben is experiencing muscular rigidity and diaphoresis. His bed linens are damp. When the nurse changes the bed, he notes that the client has been incontinent of urine and has been sweating. Ben also seems agitated and confused. His wife asks, "Do you think he might have the flu?" She explains that Ben was nauseated the day before and the family health care provider gave him a prochlorperazine (Compazine) injection and prescribed some prochlorperazine pills. She relates that Ben took twice as many pills as prescribed yet is still nauseated.

The nurse notes a fine tremor of Ben's hands after he drops a glass of water. The nurse palpates the client's abdomen and tests for rebound tenderness; then he telephones Ben's psychiatrist. The psychiatrist tells the nurse to call emergency medical services (EMS) and have Ben transported to the hospital.

Questions

1. Why did Ben's psychiatrist want him treated at the hospital instead of at home? Do all clients with signs of Neuroleptic Malignant Syndrome (NMS) need to go to the hospital for treatment? Why did the nurse test for rebound tenderness?

2. Before EMS arrives, the client's wife asks the nurse about giving the depot neuroleptic. Should the nurse give the depot neuroleptic before the client goes to the hospital? Should the nurse allow or withhold the prochlorperazine? Give a rationale for your answer.

3. What neuroleptic medications are available in depot form? How are these medications given? What medications are commonly implicated in NMS?

4. What signs and symptoms does this client have that match the criteria for the diagnosis of NMS?

5. Why must all nurses and health care providers be familiar with NMS? What is the incidence of NMS? What is the course of NMS?

6. What are the current theories on the cause(s) of NMS? What are the risk factors?

7. What teaching must be done before the client receives the first depot injection or begins taking oral neuroleptics? Beyond teaching, what else must a nurse do when working with a client who could develop NMS?

8. What is the current treatment for NMS?

9. One nurse asks, "If benztropine (Cogentin) is helpful in reducing extrapyramidal symptoms in clients whose dopamine levels are decreased by a neuroleptic, wouldn't it be helpful in treating NMS?" What answer would you give?

10. What role could this client's culture, which is a counterculture, have played in his paranoia and development of NMS? What assessments are needed in regard to culture?

11. What issues and nursing diagnoses will the visiting nurse need to work on with Ben and his wife when the NMS is resolved? What interventions would be helpful?

Questions and Suggested Answers

1. Why did Ben's psychiatrist want him treated at the hospital instead of at home? Do all clients with signs of NMS need to go to the hospital for treatment? Why did the nurse test for rebound tenderness? The psychiatrist needs to rule out various causes of this client's symptoms, including flu, acute abdomen, and NMS. The client is on a neuroleptic, has an extremely elevated temperature, and has muscle rigidity; thus, NMS is likely (APA, 2000). However, other conditions can mimic NMS. Hospitalization is recommended because NMS can be fatal. A mortality rate of 20–30 percent or greater has been associated with NMS in the recent past, but the rate is now estimated at 5–11 percent due to greater awareness, prevention, and treatment efforts (Benzer, 2005). Hospitalization facilitates performing the assessments needed to reach an accurate diagnosis. The client's mental and physical condition and blood chemistry can be monitored more closely in the hospital. Recommended blood work includes a complete blood count and serum creatine phosphokinase (CPK). Both the white blood cell (WBC) count and CPK or serum creatine kinase (CK) are typically elevated in NMS. The CPK elevation might be mild or extremely elevated. The client might need intravenous (IV) fluids and methods to lower the temperature (e.g., cooling blankets) and medications to reduce rigidity (i.e., a dopamine agonist to reverse dopamine D_2-receptor blockage). These medications include bromocriptine (Parlodel), amantadine (Symmetrel), levodopa and carbidopa (Sinemet), and dantrolene (Dantrium) (Benzer, 2005).

Most clients exhibiting signs of NMS will need the supervision, ongoing evaluation, and medications that are only available at a hospital. The most acute episodes will be treated in the intensive care unit (ICU). A client with NMS could be treated without hospitalization if signs are relatively mild and recognized early, neuroleptic medication is stopped quickly, and supportive measures are initiated.

Appendicitis often mimics NMS. Thus, the nurse tested for rebound tenderness, which typically indicates an acute appendicitis, in order to help rule out appendicitis as a cause of Ben's symptoms. *Rebound tenderness* is a sharp pain that occurs when the examiner's fingers are pressed upward and inward into the right lower quadrant and then suddenly released.

From a physiologic standpoint, this client received a depot injection that is a dopamine-blocking agent and prochlorperazine, another dopamine-blocking agent. Then, the client doubled the dose of prochlorperazine. This information, coupled with the client's age and associated decrease in dopamine levels, supports the likelihood this client is experiencing NMS.

2. Before EMS arrives, the client's wife asks about giving the depot neuroleptic. Should the nurse give the depot neuroleptic before the client goes to the hospital? Should the nurse allow or withhold the prochlorperazine? Give a rationale for your answer. The nurse must withold the injection of depot medication. If this client has NMS with depleted dopamine, giving the haloperidol decanoate injection would further deplete dopamine levels, exacerbating the symptoms and perhaps leading to death. Rosebush, Garside, and Mazurek (2004, 1645) state, "In our opinion an appropriate standard of care would necessitate immediate discontinuation of all dopamine blocking agents in probable or suspected cases [of NMS]." The client also must stop taking prochlorperazine and all other medications that have dopamine D_2-receptor antagonist properties.

3. What neuroleptic medications are available in depot form? How are these medications given? What medications are commonly implicated in NMS? Haloperidol decanoate, a high-potency drug, is one of the earliest depot forms of neuroleptics. Potency is based on a comparison with the first psychotropic or neuroleptic drug, chlorpromazine (Thorazine); only a few milligrams of haloperidol equate to 100 mg of chlorpromazine. Fluphenazine (Prolixin) decanoate is another long-acting depot neuroleptic medication. Recently, a long-acting injection form of one of the new atypical antipsychotics agents, respiradone (Risperdal), became available under the brand name Risperdal Consta. Long-acting depot neuroleptics are given deep intramuscular (IM) using the Z-Track method. It is important to aspirate before giving the medication in order to avoid injecting the medication into the bloodstream.

Benzer (2005, 2) points out that "all medications implicated in NMS have dopamine D_2-receptor antagonist properties." NMS also has occurred after withdrawal of anti-Parkinsonian medication. Potent neuroleptics such as haloperidol and fluphenazine are more often associated with NMS, but all antipsychotic (neuroleptic) medications, typical or atypical, can precipitate the syndrome. Benzer (2005) states that prochlorperazine, promethazine (Phenergan), clozapine (Clozaril), and risperidone (Risperdal) all have been associated with NMS. Other drugs that bock dopamine D_2 receptors or decrease the available dopamine but are not neuroleptics also have been implicated in NMS. These drugs include metoclopramide (Reglan), amoxapine (Asendin), and lithium.

4. What signs and symptoms does this client have that match the criteria for the diagnosis of NMS? The *Diagnostic and Statistical Manual of Mental Disorders* (APA, 2000) discusses NMS under "Criteria Sets Provided for Further Study." Its research criteria for diagnosis include elevated temperature and severe muscular rigidity as essential signs. Some clinicians describe the muscular rigidity as "lead pipe rigidity." Journal articles suggest that a client can have NMS with little or no muscle rigidity. The associated fever is often very high, rising to levels above 106°F. Some textbooks report rare cases where NMS presented with no fever (Frisch and Frisch, 2006).

The APA (2000) research criteria call for the client to have two or more of ten other signs beyond elevated temperature and muscle rigidity. The signs used to diagnose NMS must not be attributable to a neurologic or general medical condition or better explained by a mental disorder such as one with catatonic features.

Criterion for Neuroleptic Malignant Syndrome	Signs Observed in This Client
Elevated temperature	**Yes.** Has a temperature of 103°F.
Muscle rigidity	**Yes.** Has muscular rigidity.
These two symptoms above are associated with taking neuroleptic medication	**Yes.** Took haloperidol decanoate IM. Took prochlorperazine for nausea.
Must have two of the following nine symptoms	
Difficulty swallowing (dysphagia)	**No.**
Tremor	**Yes.** The nurse noted a fine tremor of the hands after the client dropped a water glass.
Incontinence	**Yes.** The nurse noted incontinence of urine when changing bed sheets.
Changes in level of consciousness	**Yes.** Client is agitated and confused.
Not speaking (mutism)	**No.**
Fast heart rate	**Yes.** The pulse was 136, which requires further assessment.
High or unstable blood pressure	**Yes.** There is one high reading, which calls for further assessment.
Leukocytosis	Needs assessment.
Laboratory clues of injury to muscle (e.g., high CPK)	Needs assessment.

5. Why must all nurses and health care providers be familiar with NMS? What is the incidence of NMS? What is the course of NMS? Although NMS is relatively rare, nurses and health care providers need to familiar with the signs of NMS because, if not treated, it can lead quickly to serious problems and death.

APA (2000) places the estimated incidence of NMS as between 0.07 percent and 1.4 percent of all individuals taking a neuroleptic medication. Waldorf (2003) offers a somewhat higher incidence rate at 0.02–3.23 percent. NMS occurs more often in males, particularly young males, although this might be due to prescribing practices that differ for males and females. Older adults are at risk for NMS due to age-associated drops in dopamine levels and other risk factors.

The signs and symptoms of NMS usually develop over a two- to three-day period and can last up to thirty days after stopping the neuroleptic medication (Waldorf, 2003). Typically, NMS resolves in five to seven days, but will take longer when a depot dopamine-blocking medication has been administered (Rosebush, Garside, and Mazurek, 2004). The client might exhibit some or all the signs and/or symptoms listed in the preceding table. In addition, oculogyric crisis, opisthotonic position (head hyperextended and body bowed), or a myocardial infarction could occur as a result of oxygen being diverted from the myocardium to skeletal muscle. The client also might develop arrhythmias. Dopamine receptor blockade in the hypothalamus can bring about alterations in vital signs (e.g., labile BP and tachycardia). In addition to mental status changes, the client can experience seizure activity. Clients with chest wall rigidity are at risk for respiratory distress and aspiration pneumonia. A client might experience myoglobulinemia and renal failure. In cases where clients have died from complications of NMS, the common causes of death were renal failure, respiratory failure, cardiac failure, and thromboembolus.

6. What are the current theories on the cause(s) of NMS? What are the risk factors? The exact cause of NMS is not known; however, clinicians operate on the theory that a deficit of dopamine causes the signs and symptoms. Neuroleptic medication is a dopamine antagonist believed to act by blocking dopamine at specific dopamine receptor sites (D_2-receptor sites), thus reducing the amount of dopamine available to circulate in the central nervous system (CNS). In NMS, it is thought that the blockade is too great and the amount of available dopamine is too small. However, not all clients develop NMS under similar circumstances. Some clients develop extrapyramidal side effects (EPSEs) when they are on neuroleptic medications, perhaps due to an imbalance of dopamine and acetylcholine.

Why do some clients develop NMS while others under similar circumstances do not? Some factors, such as age, increase the risk of NMS. Nicholson and Chiu (2004) point out that health care providers frequently prescribe neuroleptics to treat agitation in older adults who have dementia and delirium. Another risk factor is the coadministration of other dopaminergic drugs.

Some medications administered to treat nausea and vomiting or in anesthesia to prevent vomiting, such as promethazine, prochlorperazine, droperidol (Inapsine), and metoclopramide, cause a reduction in dopamine levels. Ben not only received a depot neuroleptic but also took prochlorperazine. Unlike clients who have schizophrenia or other mental disorders and have too much dopamine that must be intentionally decreased by neuroleptics, the client with Parkinson's disease lacks dopamine and must take medications such as levodopa and carbidopa and amantadine to build up dopamine levels in the CNS. It is possible that when clients who are on one of these dopamine-increasing drugs are taken off of it, they are at risk for NMS.

Risk factors include age, dehydration, medical problems, electrolyte imbalance, high-potency neuroleptic medication, depot forms of neuroleptic medication, rapid increases in dose of neuroleptic medication, and combinations of dopamine-blocking medications. Coadministration of lithium and haloperidol poses a particular risk (Waldorf, 2003).

7. What teaching must be done before the client receives the first depot injection or begins to take oral neuroleptics? Beyond teaching, what else must a nurse do when working with a client who could develop NMS? As part of the informed consent process, the nurse must provide the client and significant others a list of side effects and adverse effects, especially those that require immediate notification of the prescribing health care provider. Clients also need to know which signs and symptoms call for them to withhold the medication and notify their health care provider, such as temperatures above 101°F, rigid muscles, changes in mental alertness (mental status changes), rapid breathing, rapid heart rate, and nausea or vomiting.

The nurse also must teach clients to advise all health care providers that they are taking a neuroleptic medication and provide the type and amount of that medication. In addition, the nurse must emphasize the importance of taking all medications as prescribed and not doubling up.

Nurses and health care providers need to know about NMS because, if not treated, it can lead quickly to serious problems and even death. A nurse working with a client who is taking neuroleptic medications needs to

- Review medication instructions with the client periodically to ensure the client understands instructions, knows the signs and symptoms of side effects and adverse effects, and knows what to do when they occur.
- Monitor neuroleptic medications and question any order that suddenly increases the dose or seems excessive. In some cases, clients do require higher doses of medication, but this should be checked with the health care provider.
- Monitor concurrent orders for drugs that might cause or contribute to NMS.
- Monitor vital signs routinely and pay attention to deviations from normal.
- Maintain hydration in clients.
- Prevent exhaustion in clients.
- Monitor electrolytes in clients.

8. What is the current treatment for NMS? Initial treatment is to withhold the neuroleptic medication and any other medications that block dopamine receptors. Subsequent treatment involves giving dantrolene or other dopamine agonists, such as bromocriptine and amantadine, and providing supportive nursing actions such as hydration, cooling, and anti-thrombolytic measures. Dantrolene (Dantrium), a centrally acting skeletal muscle relaxant, is the drug most often mentioned in the literature (Nicholson and Chiu, 2004; Waldorf, 2004; Wren et al., 2003) as a treatment for NMS. Dantrolene helps ameliorate not only symptoms of muscle rigidity and resulting muscle breakdown but also the heat-generation situation (Wren et al., 2003). It is believed to release dopamine from neuronal sites where it is stored.

It might "be necessary to continue dantrolene orally with 1–2 mg/kg qid for 1–3 days to prevent reoccurrence" (Shannon, Wilson, and Stang, 2003, 417). Although dantrolene is the drug of choice of many clinicians, amantadine also is used. It is an anti-infective, antiviral, anticholinergic, and anti-Parkinsonian drug.

In some cases, electroconvulsive shock therapy and benzodiazepines are used to treat NMS. Nicholson and Chiu (2004) caution that geriatric clients might not tolerate either well; in fact, these treatments could trigger delirium.

Rosebush, Garside, and Mazurek (2004) report achieving excellent outcomes by just discontinuing the neuroleptic and initiating early supportive care. They also state there is evidence that bromocriptine prolongs the symptoms of NMS. Fekadu and Bisson (2005) caution against reinstituting a neuroleptic medication within two weeks of recovering from NMS, as this action will likely result in relapse.

9. One nurse asks, "If benztropine (Cogentin) is helpful in reducing extrapyramidal symptoms in clients whose dopamine levels are decreased by a neuroleptic, wouldn't it be helpful in treating NMS?" What answer would you give? The correct response is, "No, it is not recommended as a treatment of NMS." The physiologic basis for not giving benztropine lies in the idea that this medicine disrupts the dissipation of heat due to its ability to alter the body's normal thermoregulatory mechanism. In other words, the client with NMS typically has a fever and benztropine will help keep the temperature elevated (Waldorf, 2003).

10. What role could this client's culture, which is a counterculture, have played in his paranoia and development of NMS? What assessments are needed in regard to culture? People from anti-establishment countercultures often distrust authority figures. Taking twice as much medicine as prescribed without checking with the health care provider is a way to feel in control and snub authority. The client also might use marijuana or street drugs, both of which can cause paranoia.

The nurse must assess the client's cultural beliefs and determine how these beliefs affect his health practices and medication compliance. The nurse also must assess the client's drug use/abuse history. A drug screen is likely needed.

11. What issues and nursing diagnoses will the visiting nurse need to work on with Ben and his wife when the NMS is resolved? What interventions would be helpful? Trust is an issue, and the nurse will have to build trust and rapport with Ben and his wife. Talking on safe topics, such as motorcycles, could help build rapport. If the client remains paranoid, the nurse can teach the wife to buy foods that are canned or in unopened packages so the client will not think they are poisoned and will eat. Efforts to build trust and orient the client also will help with the nursing diagnosis, thought processes altered. Interventions might include not challenging delusions, providing a relaxing environment, and perhaps suggesting that the client listen to music.

Nursing diagnoses also will likely include social isolation as well as caregiver role strain. The nurse must work with the client to reduce isolating behavior, using his interest in motorcycles and other areas to help him set goals and increase his interactions with others. The nurse must encourage the wife to take some time for herself and activities she enjoys to recharge her energy. Also, the nurse should teach her some therapeutic communication skills.

References

American Psychiatric Association (APA). (2000). *Diagnostic and Statistical Manual of Mental Disorders, 4th ed.* Text Revision. Washington, DC: APA.

Benzer, T. I. (2005). "Neuroleptic Malignant Syndrome." www.emedicine.com/emerg/topic339.htm. Accessed May 24, 2006.

Fekadu, A. and J. I. Bisson. (2005). "Neuroleptic Malignant Syndrome: Diagnostic and Therapeutic Dilemmas." *Behavioral Neurology* 16(1): 9–13.

Frisch, N. C. and L. E. Frisch. (2006). *Psychiatric Mental Health Nursing* (2d ed.). Albany, NY: Thomson Delmar Learning.

Nicholson, D. and W. Chiu. (2004). "Neuroleptic Malignant Syndrome." *Geriatrics* 58(8): 36–40.

Rosebush, P., Garside, S., and M. F. Mazurek. (2004). "Recognizing Neuroleptic Malignant Syndrome." *Canadian Medical Association Journal* 170(11): 1645.

Shannon, M. T., Wilson, B. A., and C. L. Stang. (2003). *Prentice Hall Health Professional's Drug Guide 2003*. Upper Saddle River, NJ: Prentice Hall.

Waldorf, S. (2003). "Update for Nurse Anesthetists: Neuroleptic Malignant Syndrome." *American Association of Nurse Anesthetists Journal* 71(5): 389–94.

Wren, P., et al. (2003). "Three Potentially Adverse Effects of Psychotropic Meds." *Perspectives in Psychiatric Care* 39(2): 75–81.

PART TWO

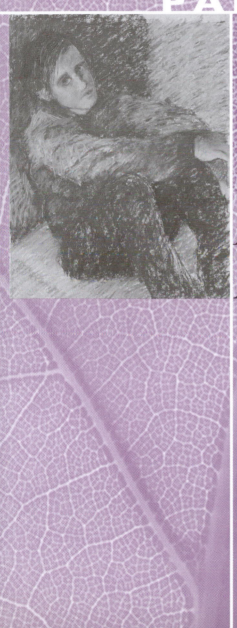

*The Client
Experiencing
Anxiety*

CASE STUDY 1

Murat

GENDER

M

AGE

14

SETTING

- School nurse's office

ETHNICITY

- Turkish American

CULTURAL CONSIDERATIONS

- Turkish

PREEXISTING CONDITION

COEXISTING CONDITION

COMMUNICATION

DISABILITY

- Obsessive-Compulsive Disorder (OCD) is a disability under the Americans with Disabilities Act (ADA)

SOCIOECONOMIC

Upper class

SPIRITUAL/RELIGIOUS

Practicing Muslim

PHARMACOLOGIC

Fluvoxamine (Luvox)

PSYCHOSOCIAL

LEGAL

- Schools must provide accommodations for disability, if needed.
- Parents must give consent to medication.

ETHICAL

- Client's right to choose and practice any religion
- The need to obtain an adolescent's consent to medication

ALTERNATIVE THERAPY

- St. John's wort and passiflora

PRIORITIZATION

DELEGATION

OBSESSIVE-COMPULSIVE DISORDER IN AN ADOLESCENT

Level of difficulty: Easy

Overview: Requires critical thinking, knowledge of the adolescent client's cultural and religious beliefs and practices, and understanding of the nursing process to determine the probable causes of reddened hands and arms and the behavior of recopying schoolwork excessively. The nurse must determine the actions to be taken.

Client Profile

Murat, a 14-year-old male, was born in Turkey, as were his parents. The family practices the Muslim faith, adhering to the required preparation for prayers and the associated rituals. When Murat was 4 years old, his family noticed he was overly concerned about his belongings not being touched and their order being maintained. He also exhibited many bedtime rituals involving hygiene issues and numbers (e.g., counting and ordering his favorite toys). As he grew older, Murat took longer and longer to complete his homework, redoing it at least once or twice. Now, Murat's preoccupation with redoing work makes it impossible for him to turn it in.

Case Study

Murat is failing several high school courses, but his parents do not know. One of Murat's teachers realizes that something must be done to help him pass his courses. She recalls seeing Murat recopying his assigned schoolwork several times before or during class. Although Murat does exceedingly well verbally in her class, the course grade is based on written work and projects, which he seldom completes or turns in. The teacher notices that Murat's hands and arms are very red; she wonders if there is a medical cause to explain this redness (e.g., an allergic reaction). The teacher also observes Murat's practice of going to the bathroom immediately after any work in pairs or groups; he also heads for the bathroom as soon as class is over. One of Murat's classmates tells the teacher that Murat feels the school is dirty and he does not like people touching him.

The teacher drops by the school nurse's office, shares her observations about Murat, and asks, "Will you look into the matter and identify how we can help him?" The nurse agrees to do so and devises a course of action. The nurse begins by developing a trusting relationship with Murat. She challenges him to a game of chess. During the game, he tells the nurse that he has tried to stop thinking about contamination and washing his hands so often, but he can't. He also says he has tried to stop recopying his papers but just can't stop feeling that they are error ridden and poorly written.

Sometime later, Murat's parents take him to see a psychiatrist who prescribes fluvoxamine (Luvox) and suggests Cognitive Behavioral Therapy (CBT).

Questions

1. If you were the nurse in this case, would you have the teacher send this student to your office or would you take a different approach?

2. Why do you think Murat avoids being touched and feels the school is dirty? How would you approach these topics with Murat?

3. Do religious rituals such as Muslim washing rituals involve obsessions and compulsions? What is an obsession? What is a compulsion?

4. Are some children's rituals considered normal? When children and adolescents have actual obsessions and compulsions, what are they like?

5. How is Obsessive-Compulsive Disorder (OCD) diagnosed? What are the criteria for OCD in a child or an adolescent?

6. What is the significance of Murat telling the nurse that he has tried to stop his thoughts about contamination and imperfection and the actions they provoke? Should the nurse develop a nursing care plan and work with Murat alone?

7. A teacher asks two questions, "What purposes do the repetitive, ritualistic, or ordering actions (compulsions) serve for this client and others with these behaviors?" and "Should Murat be prevented from carrying out compulsions?" How would you respond?

8. What treatments is the psychiatrist likely to suggest if Murat is diagnosed with OCD or is seen to manifest OCD traits?

9. After consulting the psychiatrist, Murat's mother asks about the efficacy of a herbal remedy she saw advertised on the Internet as a treatment for OCD. The main ingredients are passiflora and St. John's wort. What would you tell her?

10. Murat's parents are reluctant to sign a consent form allowing Murat to take fluvoxamine (Luvox) or any selective serotonin reuptake inhibitor (SSRI). You feel strongly about this treatment. What would you say or do?

11. Murat and his parents ask about the causes of OCD. They also ask about PANDAS. How would you answer their questions? What is PANDAS?

12. What are the likely nursing diagnoses and goals? What interventions would be helpful?

Questions and Suggested Answers

1.   If you were the nurse in this case, would you have the teacher send this student to your office or would you take a different approach? Unless you have an established relationship with Murat or he is an exceptionally open adolescent, it would not be productive to send for him and ask about what is going on. Being summoned can make a person anxious and guarded. You first need to devise a nonthreatening way to interact with Murat and build some trust and rapport before probing about his reddened skin. One idea involves visiting Murat's classroom, having the teacher introduce you, and giving a short presentation in which you involve Murat. This positive interaction will not only build his self-esteem but also show you as an empathic person. You could make a point of seeing him a short while later, reintroducing yourself, and asking him to stop by your office for a few minutes so you can get his ideas on some matter.

When broaching the subject of his reddened hands and arms, you must use therapeutic communication techniques. You could make an observation such as, "I notice your hands and arms are red" and wait until he responds. The objective is to be as nonthreatening as possible using an open-ended technique that does not lead the client.

2. Why do you think Murat avoids being touched and feels the school is dirty? How would you approach these topics with Murat? Perfectly normal people often refuse to drink from a water fountain after seeing people touch their mouths to the fountain spigot. Others use a paper towel to turn off lavatory faucets rather than their bare hands; many more avoid shaking hands due to germs. In fact, many cultures do not shake hands. For example, Asians bow from the waist or put the palms of their hands together with fingers pointed up and bow their head in a sign of greeting. Thus, culture could account for Murat's aversion to shaking hands; however, it could involve an obsession and compulsion as well.

While OCD could account for his frequent trips to the bathroom and the redness of his hands and arms, other possible explanations exist. Anyone familiar with the Muslim religion knows there are washing rituals before prayers known as *wudu*; perhaps, the soap Murat uses to execute these extensive rituals irritates his skin (www.islamonline.net/english/introducingislam/Worship/Prayers/article01.shtml, 2005).

3. Do religious rituals such as Muslim washing rituals involve obsessions and compulsions? What is an obsession? What is a compulsion? *Obsessions* are "recurrent and persistent thoughts, impulses, or images that the person finds at some time during the disturbance to be intrusive and inappropriate and that cause marked distress or anxiety" (APA, 2000, 462). *Compulsions* are repetitive behaviors, such as checking, counting, ordering, and washing, or acts of the mind, such as repeating words or counting or praying silently, that an individual feels compelled to do in response to an obsessive thought or according to rigid rules (APA, 2000).

When religious rituals do not cause an individual distress, the idea of performing them is not considered an obsession and the rituals themselves are not considered compulsions. When thoughts of performing religious rituals become intrusive and the person cannot stop these thoughts or performs the rituals so often that they cause problems in the person's life, then the person likely has religious obsessions and compulsions.

Okasha (2004) reports on the effects of the Egyptian culture and the Muslim religion on Egyptian adolescents with OCD. He estimates the incidence as approximately 2.5 percent, adding, "religion and prevailing traditions seemed to color not only the clinical picture of the condition [OCD] but also the patient's attitudes about the disorder" (Okasha, 2004, 21). He identifies religion, contamination, and somatic complaints as the most common obsessions in this cultural group.

4. Are some children's rituals considered normal? When children and adolescents have actual obsessions and compulsions, what are they like? Children normally engage in "just right" and repetitive types of compulsivity to help master anxiety and exercise some degree of control over their ever-changing environment. Wigren and Hansen (2003) report that normal compulsivity typically reaches a peak at age 4.

When children manifest true obsessions and compulsions, they are similar to those experienced by adults but reflect the child's developmental level. Younger children tend to have concrete types of rituals (e.g., intrusive thoughts that something bad has happened to, or will happen to, their primary caregiver [usually mother] or someone close to them and that the threat results from their behavior or thinking). All children periodically experience these feelings, as do many adults. These thoughts become problematic when they persist and interfere with their school or home life. Children can take on responsibility for keeping someone safe by repeatedly checking to see whether windows and doors are locked or performing rituals they believe will neutralize the danger.

As children learn to count, they might realize it takes a given number of steps to reach a certain place or that they touch things in certain ways or a given number of times. This counting behavior is normal unless it persists and interferes with the child's life.

Older children might spend hours rewriting papers to ensure they are perfect. Likewise, they might be obsessed with germs and wash excessively, avoid contamination, or perform rituals to undo contact with someone or something perceived to be "dirty." Adolescents can have multiple obsessions and/or compulsions.

Rapoport (1990) categorizes obsessions as aggressive; contamination; and need for symmetry, exactness, or order obsessions. She categorizes compulsions as somatic; counting; checking; repeating rituals; ordering/arranging rituals; hoarding/collecting; and miscellaneous compulsions (need to tell, ask, or confess; need to touch or measure).

5. How is OCD diagnosed? What are the criteria for OCD in a child or an adolescent? The qualified professional starts by taking a complete family history and looking for a history of relatives with OCD and Tourette's syndrome, which is often associated with OCD. Next, the diagnostician tries to determine whether the child's signs or symptoms are consistent with OCD diagnostic criteria. The diagnostic instrument of choice is the Yale-Brown Obsessive-Compulsive Scale (Tynan, 2005, 4; Stein, 2002, 400).

Regardless of client age, a diagnosis of OCD requires that the following criteria be met:

- The client must exhibit either obsessions or compulsions (or both).
- The obsessions must go beyond mere worry about real-life problems.
- The individual must try to ignore the obsession or stop it by focusing on another thought or action.
- The individual must realize that the obsessional cognitions, impulses, or images originate in his or her mind.
- The compulsive behaviors or acts must seek to avoid or reduce distress or prevent the occurrence of a dreaded happening or situation, yet there is no realistic connection between the behavior or act and the event it is supposed to neutralize or prevent or the act or behavior is excessive (APA, 2000).

A *Diagnostic and Statistical Manual of Mental Disorders* (APA, 2000) criterion requires that adults recognize that their obsessions or compulsions are excessive or unreasonable. While not a requirement for children, some do recognize the senselessness of their obsessions or compulsions or eventually come to understand this through therapy. The *Harvard Mental Health Letter* (2002, 5) points out "even young children often know that their obsessions are senseless, but they are helpless to stop themselves."

6. What is the significance of Murat telling the nurse that he has tried to stop his thoughts about contamination and imperfection and the actions they provoke? Should the nurse develop a nursing care plan and work with Murat alone? This information provides another clue that Murat is having obsessions and compulsions. It also suggests he trusts the nurse and is ready to be helped. The nurse should not work alone with Murat. This problem exceeds a school nurse's scope. Collaboration, perhaps in the form of a joint meeting with school psychologists, teachers, and parents, is indicated. Some initial steps for helping Murat might result (e.g., buying a milder soap; breaking written school assignments into smaller segments, etc.). Moreover, holding a meeting communicates to the parents the shared desire to help Murat succeed in school. In addition, it serves as a means to ascertain the parents' opinions and identify their actions to date. It also might reveal any reluctance on their part to take Murat to a child psychiatrist for evaluation.

7. A teacher asks two questions, "What purposes do the repetitive, ritualistic, or ordering actions (compulsions) serve for this client and others with these behaviors?" and "Should Murat be prevented from carrying out compulsions?" How would you respond? Compulsions serve to relieve anxiety and tension. Persons often use compulsions to neutralize a thought, prevent impulse execution, and/or prevent something awful from happening.

Frisch and Frisch (2006, 201) state, "Do not take away the compulsive rituals (unless they are dangerous) until the client has some other method in place to deal with the anxiety." Using CBT, the therapist can systematically and therapeutically help the client delay obsessions and compulsions or shorten the time spent on them (see suggested answer to question 8 below).

8. What treatments is the psychiatrist likely to suggest if Murat is diagnosed with OCD or is seen to manifest OCD traits? According to Tynan (2005), CBT and pharmacotherapy work well together clinically. Many clinicians believe that most children with OCD benefit from the combined treatment. Others (Pediatric OCD Treatment Study [POTS] Team, 2004) recommend a combination of a particular SSRI and CBT or CBT alone.

Some parents oppose medication use in children and adolescents in general; other opposition arises from a warning by the U.S. Food and Drug Administration (FDA) that the use of antidepressants in children and teenagers, as well as adults, can worsen depression and increase the risk of suicide or self injury (FDA, 2004).

Six drugs show efficacy in treating OCD clients of all ages (*Harvard Mental Health Letter*, 2002). Five are SSRIs: fluoxetine (Prozac), sertraline (Zoloft), paroxetine (Paxil), fluvoxamine (Luvox), and citalopram (Celexa). Fluvoxamine was the first SSRI to be approved by the FDA for treatment of OCD in children and adolescents. Previously, clomipramine (Anafranil), a tricyclic antidepressant, was the FDA-approved drug for children age 10 and older. It is now a second-line drug for treatment of OCD and carries some risk for adverse cardiac effects (Ables et al., 2003). Clients typically require at least two months on medication to see a decrease in symptoms; however, Sallinen and colleagues (2004) report remarkable results with clomipramine and fluoxetine followed by manual-based CBT. This regimen greatly reduced the number of obsessions and avoidance behaviors and, after three sessions of CBT, the medication was tapered and withdrawn.

One source (NIMH, 2003) states that traditional psychotherapy with the goal of client insight is usually not helpful for the client with OCD and suggests that a specific behavior therapy approach, Exposure and Response Prevention (E/RP), is more effective. This technique, which requires special therapist training, calls for clients to confront any ideas or objects they fear either directly or using their imagination (e.g., having the client touch a dirty object and resist hand washing for a prescribed period of time). The therapist encourages the client to refrain from ritualizing. With repetition, the urge to carry out compulsions diminishes. In addition to E/RP, which is part of the behavioral treatment in CBT, there is a cognitive component wherein the client learns how to identify irrational ideas and change them. Parents are integral to the success of CBT and often help with CBT homework assignments.

9. After consulting the psychiatrist, Murat's mother asks about the efficacy of a herbal remedy she saw advertised on the Internet as a treatment for OCD. The main ingredients are passiflora and St. John's wort. What would you tell her? The best approach is to demonstrate an interest in the advertisement and promise to review it. Then you should stress the importance of never taking or giving herbal remedies without first checking with a health care provider due to the possibility of drug interactions or side effects. You also could mention that herbal preparations such as passiflora and St. John's wort have not been proven to be effective treatment for children and adolescents with OCD. You should advise her to call the psychiatrist who prescribed the fluvoxamine before administering this herbal preparation to Murat.

10. Murat's parents are reluctant to sign a consent form allowing Murat to take fluvoxamine or any SSRI. You feel strongly about this treatment. What would you say or do? You could provide research findings on the use of SSRIs, both pro and con. You also could ask the parents to list their reasons for and against the medication and respond to their concerns. And you could suggest they discuss it further with the psychiatrist, stay open to the possibility, and continue to look for updated information. You cannot ethically push your choice on the parents. You can advise them on the importance of educating adolescents about the medication, requesting their opinion, and asking them to sign a consent for medication along with the parents. Seeking adolescents' consent promotes the idea of their being in control and helps increase compliance with the medication regimen.

11. Murat and his parents ask about the causes of OCD. They also ask about PANDAS. How would you answer their questions? What is PANDAS? The causes of OCD are unknown, but there is probably a hereditary and a neurobiologic component. A growing body of evidence supports the neurobiologic basis; in particular, brain imaging studies reveal greater activity in the frontal cortex when OCD is present (Sallinen, 2002, 5). Serotonin probably plays a role in OCD, as SSRIs are effective in reducing obsessions and/or compulsions. OCD tends to run in families.

Researchers (Murphy and Pichichero, 2002) propose a condition called pediatric autoimmune neuropsychiatry disorders associated with streptococcal infections (PANDAS) as a cause of OCD in a small subset of children age three to puberty. Proponents believe that OCD might be associated with Group A beta-hemolytic streptococcal infections (GABHS), for example, scarlet fever and "strep" throat. This type of OCD is often associated with neurologic abnormalities, such as tics and choreiform movements.

Kurlan and Kaplan (2004), among others, question this theory, saying it is an unproven hypothesis. Other research (Luo et al., 2004) showed no or insufficient evidence to support the assertion that GABHS causes or exacerbates OCD. GABHS is common in the upper respiratory tract of school-age children who are asymptomatic. Further, many adolescents with OCD had obsessions and compulsions early in childhood, but they were not recognized as such. Moreover, symptoms tend to wax and wane, becoming worse under stress such as an infection.

12. What are the likely nursing diagnoses and goals? What interventions would be helpful? Nursing diagnoses include, but are not limited to, anxiety; powerlessness; ineffective coping, deficient diversional activity (needs further assessment); impaired skin integrity.

Goals could include:

Identify at least one appropriate way to reduce anxiety.
Effect a noticeable reduction in redness of hands and arms.
Demonstrate the use of at least two effective coping mechanisms.
Engage in at least one diversional activity that reduces his anxiety.

Interventions likely to be helpful include:

- Model and teach relaxation techniques.
- Model and teach decision-making skills.
- Model and teach recognition and correction of thinking errors.
- Provide support to the family.
- Provide liaison between the school and the family.
- Provide a listening person for the student and family.
- Offer positive reinforcement for the student and family for any progress toward meeting goals.
- Include the student and family as part of the team.
- Help the student find areas and ways in which to excel.
- Help the student identify future goals.
- Facilitate opportunities for the student to interact positively with peers and make friends.
- Monitor and facilitate cleanliness in bathrooms.

References

Ables, A. Z., et al. (2003). Antidepressants; Update on New Agents and Indications. *American Family Physician* 67: 547–555.

American Psychiatric Association (APA). (2000). *Diagnostic and Statistical Manual of Mental Disorders, 4th ed.* Text Revision. Washington, DC: APA.

FDA. (2004). FDA Talk Paper: FDA Issues Public Health Advisory on Cautions for Use of Antidepressants in Adults and Children, www.fda.gov/bbs/topics/ANSWERS/2004/ANSO1283.html.

Frisch, N. C. and L. E. Frisch. (2006). *Psychiatric Mental Health Nursing, 3d ed.* Albany, NY: Thomson Delmar Learning.

IOL Team. (2003). "Conditions of Prayer: Physical Purity." www.islamonline.net/english/introducingislam/Worship/Prayers/article01.shtml. Accessed May 29, 2006.

Kurlan R. and E. L. Kaplan. (2004). "The Pediatric Autoimmune Neuropsychiatric Disorders Associated with Streptococcal Infection (PANDAS) Etiology for Tics and Obsessive-Compulsive Symptoms: Hypothesis or Entity? Practical Considerations for the Clinician." *Pediatrics* 113(4): 883–887.

Luo, F., et al. (2004). "Prospective Longitudinal Study of Children with Tic Disorders and/or Obsessive-Compulsive Disorder: Relationship of Symptom Exacerbations to Newly Acquired Streptococcal Infections." *Pediatrics* 113(6): 578–584.

Murphy, M. L. and M. E. Pichichero. (2002). "Prospective Identification and Treatment of Children with Pediatric Autoimmune Neuropsychiatric Disorder Associated with Group A Streptococcal Infection (PANDAS)." *Archives of Pediatrics and Adolescent Medicine* 156: 356–361.

NIMH. (2003). "Obsessive-Compulsive Disorder." www.nimh.nih.gov/publicat/ocd.cfm. Accessed November 28, 2003.

"Obsessions and Compulsions in Children." (2002). *Harvard Mental Health Letter* 19: 4–9.

Okasha, A. (2004). "OCD in Egyptian Adolescents: The Effect of Culture and Religion." *Psychiatric Times* (April, Special ed.): 21(5): 21–22.

Pediatric OCD Treatment Study (POTS) Team. "Cognitive-Behavior Therapy, Sertraline, and Their Combination for Children and Adolescents with Obsessive-Compulsive Disorder: The Pediatric OCD Treatment Study (POTS) Randomized Controlled Trial." (2004). *Journal of the American Medical Association* 292(16): 1969–1976.

Rapoport, J. L. (1990). *The Boy Who Couldn't Stop Washing: The Experience and Treatment of Obsessive-Compulsive Disorder.* New York: Penguin Putnam Inc.

Sallinen, B. J., et al. (2004). "Case Study: Successful Medication Withdrawal Using Cognitive-Behavioral Therapy for a Preadolescent with OCD." *Journal of the American Academy of Child Adolescent Psychiatry* 43(11): 1441–1444.

Stein, D. J. (2002). "Obsessive-Compulsive Disorder." *Lancet* 360 (9330): 397–406.

Tynan, W. D. (2005). "Discussion of Anxiety Disorder: Obsessive Compulsive Disorder." www.emedicine.com/ped/topic2794.htm. Accessed June 27, 2005.

Wigren, M. and S. Hansen. (2003). "Rituals and Compulsivity in Prader-Willi Syndrome: Profile and Stability." *Journal of Intellectual Disability Research* 47(6): 428–437.

CASE STUDY 2

Alyssa

GENDER

F

AGE

25

SETTING

■ Medical clinic

ETHNICITY

■ White American

CULTURAL CONSIDERATIONS

■ Spouse is Hispanic (Puerto Rican)

PREEXISTING CONDITION

COEXISTING CONDITION

COMMUNICATION

DISABILITY

SOCIOECONOMIC

SPIRITUAL/RELIGIOUS

■ Catholic

PHARMACOLOGIC

■ Fluvoxamine (Luvox)

PSYCHOSOCIAL

LEGAL

■ Confidentiality

ETHICAL

ALTERNATIVE THERAPY

■ Behavior therapy

PRIORITIZATION

DELEGATION

MODERATE

OBSESSIVE COMPULSIVE DISORDER

Level of difficulty: Moderate

Overview: Requires the nurse to be knowledgeable about Obsessive-Compulsive Disorder (OCD) and to apply critical thinking in working effectively with a client who has signs and symptoms of this disorder and her husband. The nurse must gain an understanding of the husband's culture-driven behavior.

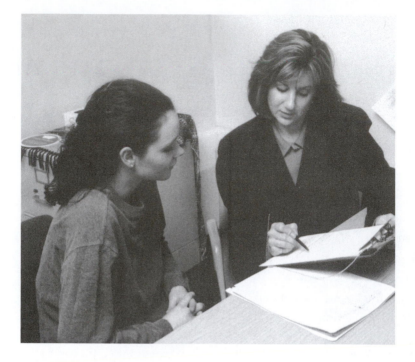

Client Profile

Alyssa is a 25-year-old female whose husband is Puerto Rican. About eight years ago, Alyssa began washing her hands repeatedly. She also started showering several times a day. About one year ago, she began checking the door locks over and over, unable to go to bed or to leave home until she checked them three hundred or more times. Over the past few months, these behaviors have escalated. Her husband is upset that Alyssa does not come to bed when he does.

Alyssa cannot throw away cardboard boxes, magazines, or plastic bottles. Her house and garage are cluttered with items she is saving in case she might need them. The car cannot be parked in the garage because there is no room.

Case Study

Alyssa presents at the medical clinic for an annual checkup. Her husband, Ricardo, accompanies her. The nurse wants to do an assessment before the physical, but Alyssa says she must wash her hands. When Alyssa returns, the nurse attempts to shake her hand; Alyssa draws away, takes out a wet wipe, and cleans her hands. The nurse says, "I notice your hands are quite red." Alyssa replies, "I guess I am washing my hands too much. I try not to wash so often, but I just can't stop." The husband tells the nurse the number of times his wife washes her hands every day, how many showers she takes, and how she rechecks the door locks three hundred or more times. Ricardo follows his wife to the examination room.

During the history taking, the husband finishes answers for his wife, indicating she has no health problems and is taking only a daily vitamin with iron. The nurse asks the client if she has anything to add, but she shakes her head. The nurse asks Ricardo, "How would you like the health care provider to help you and your wife?" The husband replies, "I would like my wife to come to bed with me instead of checking door locks. We are never intimate any more. I wonder if I should drag her to bed and hold her there." The husband, who is standing close to the nurse and gesturing with his hands and face, makes the nurse uncomfortable; she takes a step back and says, "We will talk about that later. Thank you for your help; please return to the waiting room." The client tells the nurse that her husband is angry because she will not get rid of anything. She adds, "My bedroom floor is covered with boxes full of things I am saving. It is hard to find a path to the bed."

The nurse asks Alyssa, "Do you ever have unwanted thoughts that seem to repeat themselves?" Alyssa responds, "Yes, I am afraid someone will hurt me and my husband. I think about germs that will make me sick. I am also afraid I will lose control during Mass and take off all my clothes."

The nurse asks Alyssa if she knows what is causing the repeated hand washing, showering, door checking, and intrusive thoughts in church. Alyssa admits to having had a brief affair with a married man when she was in high school. She thinks the stress of keeping this event secret, coupled with guilt, is causing her symptoms.

After the health care provider examines the client, orders some laboratory testing including a pregnancy test and a drug screen, and checks for various conditions, he writes a tentative diagnosis of Obsessive-Compulsive Disorder (OCD) and prescribes fluvoxamine (Luvox), an anti-obsession and antidepressant medication. He refers the client for individual therapy with an advanced practice nurse, a psychiatric/mental health clinical specialist who works with clients who have OCD.

Questions

1. What is an obsession? What is a compulsion? What obsessions and compulsions does this client manifest? What are some common obsessions and compulsions found in clients with OCD?

2. What criteria would Alyssa have to meet to have a diagnosis of OCD? Does she have behaviors that match these criteria? Is she aware that her obsessions and compulsions are irrational?

3. What purposes do the repetitive, ritualistic, or ordering actions (compulsions) serve for clients with these behaviors?

4. The husband asks if he should "drag his wife to bed and hold her there," implying a desire to take action to stop her from checking the door repeatedly. Should the client be prevented from carrying out compulsions?

5. How well did the nurse handle the situation when the husband was close to her, making gestures and talking about the lack of sex with his wife? What was behind his actions? Recall how he finished sentences for his wife. Was he being "macho" or is there another explanation?

6. What are the age of onset, the male-to-female ratio, and the prevalence of OCD?

7. Alyssa reports that her obsessive-compulsive behaviors began eight years ago, yet she is just now seeking help. Is this time lag unusual? Why might Alyssa have waited this long? Why is she seeking help now?

8. Would it be a good idea for the nurse to ask the husband to step out during the initial history and nursing assessment as well as the physical examination by the health care provider?

9. What laboratory tests and screens should the health care provider order/do for a client with a tentative diagnosis of OCD?

10. What is the current thinking about the etiology of OCD?

11. What is the current treatment for OCD?

12. If you were the nurse in this case, what teaching would you do for the client and her husband about fluvoxamine?

13. The health care provider refers this client to a psychiatric/mental health nurse practitioner. Do you think this is a good idea? If so, why? To what other professionals could this client be referred?

Questions and Suggested Answers

1. What is an obsession? What is a compulsion? What obsessions and compulsions does this client manifest? What are some common obsessions and compulsions found in clients with OCD? An *obsession* is a repeated (persistent) idea, thought, image, and/or impulse that is intrusive, inappropriate, and unwanted and causes a person to have excessive anxiety or distress. A *compulsion* is a repeated physical (such as washing and checking) or mental (such as silently repeating words) action that consumes a lot of time or causes significant distress or impairment that is performed to prevent or reduce anxiety or distress.

This client's obsessions involve repeated thoughts about washing her hands and body, checking the doors, and taking off her clothes in church.

Her compulsions are the actual repeated incidences of hand washing, showering, and checking doors as well as hoarding (Seedat and Stein, 2002).

Compulsions tend to fall under the following categories (NIMH 1999, 2000):

- *Cleaning*—Hand-washing rituals or repeatedly cleaning household surfaces
- *Repeating*—Uttering a name or phrase or executing a behavior over and over
- *Completing*—Performing series of complicated behaviors in exact order (i.e., rituals)
- *Checking*—Repeatedly checking items such as locks or appliances to see if they are locked or turned off
- *Being meticulous*—Overwhelming concern about where to place things in a room or its overall appearance
- *Hoarding*—Saving or collecting things of no value and being unable to dispose of them no matter how much difficulty or distress the clutter brings
- *Slowness*—Doing tasks very slowly

2. What criteria would Alyssa have to meet to have a diagnosis of OCD? Does she have behaviors that match these criteria? Is she aware that her obsessions and compulsions are irrational? To meet the diagnostic criteria of the *Diagnostic and Statistical Manual of Mental Disorders* (APA, 2000), a person must have either obsessions or compulsions. Alyssa has both. The obsessions or compulsions must be recurrent and persistent, experienced at some time as being unwanted and inappropriate, and the source of significant anxiety and distress. The adult client must recognize that the obsessions and/or compulsions are excessive or not reasonable. They must cause excessive distress, absorb one or more hours a day, or significantly interfere one or more of the client's usual routine, occupational functioning, social activities, and/or relationships (APA, 2000).

Alyssa's hand washing is recurrent, persistent, and unwanted. Her husband is distressed about some of her compulsions, especially her hoarding and those behaviors that prevent her from being available for sexual intimacy. Alyssa might be more distressed about other obsessions and compulsions, especially her inability to stop washing her hands and the struggle not to take off her clothes at Mass. The obsessions and compulsions interfere with her relationship with her husband and consume more than one hour a day. They likely interfere with her ability to enjoy or participate fully in Mass.

Obsessions must be more than excessive worry about real problems, and the adult client must recognize that the obsessions and/or compulsions are a product of her own mind. The obsessions and/or compulsions cannot result from another disorder (e.g., a preoccupation with food in an eating disorder) or alcohol consumption. While the health care provider must rule out other disorders and alcohol abuse, Alyssa appears to meet the criteria for OCD.

Notably, children do not need to recognize their obsessions or compulsions as excessive or unreasonable in order to be diagnosed with OCD. The *Harvard Mental Health Letter* (2002, 4) points out, "even young children often know that their obsessions are senseless, but they are helpless to stop themselves."

3. What purposes do the repetitive, ritualistic, or ordering actions (compulsions) serve for clients with these behaviors? Compulsions relieve anxiety and tension. Clients use compulsions to neutralize thoughts, prevent themselves from carrying out impulses, and/or prevent something awful from happening. Alyssa possesses insight into the possible source of her anxiety: the sexual affair with a married man when she was in high school. Her Catholic upbringing tells her this is a sin. Tension might arise from guilt and efforts to keep the affair secret from her husband.

4. The husband asks if he should "drag his wife to bed and hold her there," implying a desire to take action to stop her from checking the door repeatedly. Should the client be prevented from carrying out compulsions? Psychiatric texts instruct nurses and other health care providers not to stop a client's compulsions, unless they are dangerous to the client or others, until the client possesses other means to reduce anxiety (Frisch and Frisch, 2006). The nurse must explain this construct to the husband, stressing the importance of supporting his wife in following the treatment regimen.

5. How well did the nurse handle the situation when the husband was close to her, making gestures and talking about the lack of sex with his wife? What was behind his actions? Recall how he finished sentences for his wife. Was he being "macho" or is there another explanation? The husband is Puerto Rican, a country with a culture that reflects a rich mix of ethnic groups including Spanish, Taino Indian, Italian, French, German, Cuban, and American. The people of Puerto Rico tend to interrupt each other often and finish sentences for each other; such actions are accepted practice. The culture calls for a much closer social distance than in the United States or Europe. In fact, moving away from someone standing close to you is considered offensive or insulting in this culture (Rivera, 2006). The nurse must explain to the client's husband that she is not comfortable standing so close to someone and request that he keep an arm's length distance. Otherwise, she must work on developing tolerance for someone standing so close during conversation. While the husband might possess some macho traits, he just as easily might not.

6. What are the age of onset, the male-to-female ratio, and the prevalence of OCD? OCD usually begins in adolescence or early adulthood; however, it is found in children, adolescents, and adults. The *Harvard Mental Health Letter* (2002) points out that of the 2–3 percent of Americans with OCD, between one-third and one-half are under age 15; however, symptoms can appear in some children as early as age three. OCD affects more boys than girls in childhood, while it affects men and women equally in adulthood. Stein (2002) relates that OCD was once thought to be a rare condition, but it is now seen as one of the more prevalent and disabling psychiatric disorders. The *Diagnostic and Statistical Manual of Mental Disorders* (APA, 2002, 460) gives the lifetime prevalence as 2.5 percent, which means that about one adult in forty will be affected sometime in their lifetime. OCD is more prevalent than schizophrenia and bipolar disorder. Prevalence rates are similar in different cultures throughout the world.

7. Alyssa reports that her obsessive-compulsive behaviors began eight years ago, yet she is just now seeking help. Is this time lag unusual? Why might Alyssa have waited this long? Why is she seeking help now? Hollander and associates (1997) found a lag time of seventeen years from symptom onset to diagnosis of OCD in the adult clients in their study. Thus, Alyssa's lag time is not unusual. People with OCD symptoms might conceal their symptoms out of embarrassment, be unaware of available help, think they cannot afford help, or feel they can control their symptoms eventually. Alyssa's husband is prompting her help-seeking behaviors because his needs are not being met and because he is concerned about her well-being.

8. Would it be a good idea for the nurse to ask the husband to step out during the initial brief history and nursing assessment as well as the physical examination by the health care provider? Yes, it is a good idea. This way, the nurse is preserving a time in which the client can discuss things she does not want her husband to know, or know yet. In so doing, the nurse lets the client know that she still possesses control over what she shares with her husband and when she shares it. This could pose an ethical issue for nurses who believe that spouses must not have secrets.

9. What laboratory tests and screens should the health care provider order/do for a client with a tentative diagnosis of OCD? The health care provider should order a drug screen, check for signs and symptoms of Tourette's syndrome, ask about other medical and mental disorders, especially depression, inquire about drug and alcohol abuse, and ask about the client's history of streptococcal infections. This approach allows the health care provider to rule out physiologic effects of a substance or a general medical condition. The health care provider cannot reach a diagnosis of OCD until such conditions have been eliminated.

OCD symptoms sometimes occur after the administration of dopamine agonists such as methylphenidate or cocaine; notably, neurologic lesions of the cortico-striatal-thalmic-cortical circuits have been identified. If Alyssa had admitted to another psychiatric disorder, the health care provider would have to determine if the content of the obsessions or compulsions is restricted to that disorder. For example, if Alyssa had a major depressive disorder and guilt thoughts or an eating disorder and intrusive thoughts and repetitive behaviors revolving around food, the diagnosis of OCD could not be made.

The tics associated with Tourette's syndrome are not considered compulsions; however, OCD can occur concurrently in people with Tourette's syndrome. The health care provider must ask about streptococcal infection because a subset of children develops OCD after such an infection, giving rise to the possibly of an autoimmune basis. Depression often accompanies OCD (Mascltis et al., 2003).

10. What is the current thinking about the etiology of OCD? The cause of OCD is unknown. However, research using brain imaging indicates that clients with OCD possess structural and functional differences in their brains, including abnormalities such as "decreased volume or increased grey matter density in cortico-straital-thalamic-cortical circuits" (Stein, 2002, 400). Imaging also demonstrates that OCD is characterized by "increased activity in orbitofrontal cortex, cingulated, and striatum at rest," especially when exposed to feared stimuli (Stein, 2002, 400). Symptoms of OCD occur in some neurologic disorders with striatal involvement, including Tourette's syndrome, Parkinson's disease, Sydenham's chorea, and Huntington's chorea (Stein, 2002, 400). Some selective serotonin reuptake inhibitors (SSRIs) are effective in treating OCD suggesting that serotonin plays a role in OCD.

11. What is the current treatment for OCD? The literature supports a combination of medication and behavior therapy. The *Harvard Mental Health Letter* (2002) discusses six drugs, five of which are SSRIs, that show efficacy in treating OCD in children and adults: fluoxetine (Prozac), sertraline (Zoloft), paroxetine (Paxil), fluvoxamine (Luvox), citalopram (Celexa), and clomipramine (Anafranil). SSRIs are considered safer and have fewer side effects.

Both fluvoxamine and clomipramine treat obsessions as well as depression; however, clomipramine causes irregular heart rhythms and elevated blood pressure in some clients. Thus, periodic heart monitoring is necessary when it is prescribed. Clients require at least two months on medication before a decrease in symptoms occurs. The rate of improvement in clients taking medication for OCD and those receiving behavior therapy is high. Symptoms might be relieved, but they are rarely eliminated (Ables et al., 2003).

Traditional psychotherapy with the goal of client insight is usually not helpful in clients with OCD; instead, a specific behavior therapy approach—exposure and response prevention (ERP)—is more likely to be effective (NIMH, 1999). This approach, which requires special training, calls for clients to confront the ideas or objects they fear, either directly or via their imagination. Concurrently, the therapist encourages the client to refrain from ritualizing (e.g., having the client touch a dirty object and resist hand washing or cleaning for a specified period of time). With repetition, the urge to carry out compulsions diminishes because the client builds learns to resist thoughts, a behavior reinforced when nothing bad happens as a result.

12. If you were the nurse in this case, what teaching would you do for the client and her husband about fluvoxamine? Teaching should communicate the following information:

1. You must take the medication for approximately two months before improvements will occur; do not become discouraged if no changes in thinking and/or behavior happen before that time.
2. You must not abruptly stop taking the medication. Your dosage will be adjusted upward to the therapeutic level; then you will be tapered off the medication.
3. You must report any side effects or problems to the nurse or the prescribing health care provider.
4. You should avoid driving or using machinery until you are sure that the medication does not impair judgment or adversely affect motor skills.
5. You should avoid alcohol and monoamine oxidase (MAO) inhibitors as they can cause serious drug interactions. You should report any over-the-counter medications you are taking, as some can cause drug interactions.
6. You should notify your health care provider if you are pregnant or planning to become pregnant or breast feeding or planning to breast feed. This medication might be harmful to the fetus or might be carried in the mother's milk and be harmful to the baby.
7. You should report any suicidal ideation, as this medication might increase the risk of suicidal ideation.

13. The health care provider refers this client to a psychiatric/mental health nurse practitioner. Do you think this is a good idea? If so, why? To what other professionals could this client be referred? The health care provider could refer the client to a psychiatrist, a psychotherapist, or a psychologist. There is an advantage to being referred to a psychiatric/ mental health nurse practitioner: this nurse usually works closely with a psychiatrist who can prescribe medication or, if the nurse has prescribing privileges, can recommend medications. If properly trained, the psychiatric/ mental health nurse practitioner also can deliver ERP therapy and other appropriate treatments.

Psychotherapists possess a variety of educational and training backgrounds including social work, professional counseling, and nursing. They should have a license and credentials. Psychiatrists most often do psychiatric evaluation and medication prescription and management. They often do not provide behavior therapy. Psychologists do not prescribe. Referral to a psychologist is helpful when psychological testing is needed.

References

Ables, A. Z., et al. (2003). "Antidepressants; Update on New Agents and Indications." *American Family Physician* 67: 547–555.

American Psychiatric Association (APA). (2000). *Diagnostic and Statistical Manual of Mental Disorders, 4th ed.* Text Revision. Washington, DC: APA.

Frisch, N. C. and L. E. Frisch. (2006). *Psychiatric Mental Health Nursing, 2d ed.* Albany, NY: Thompson Delmar Learning.

Hollander, E., et al. (1997). "A Pharmacoeconomic and Quality of Life Study of Obsessive-Compulsive Disorder." *CNS Spectrum* 2: 16–25.

Mascltis, M., et al. (2003). "Quality of Life in OCD: Differential Impact of Obsessions, Compulsions, and Depression Comorbidity." *Canadian Journal of Psychiatry* 48: 72–77.

National Institute of Mental Health (NIMH). (1999). "Facts About Obsessive-Compulsive Disorder." Bethesda, MD: NIMH, National Institutes of Health. http://www.nimh.nih.gov/publicat/ocdfacts.pdf. Accessed December 2003.

——. (2000). *Obsessive-Compulsive Disorder (OCD), A Real Illness.* Bethesda, MD: NIMH, National Institutes of Health. Available at www.nimh.nih.gov/publicat/ NIMHocd.pdf. Accessed June 2, 2006.

"Obsessions and Compulsions in Children." (2002). *Harvard Mental Health Letter* 19(1): 4–7.

Rivera, M. (2006). "Puerto Rican Culture." http://welcome.topuertorico.org/culture. Accessed May 25, 2006.

Seedat, S. and D. J. Stein. (2002). "Hoarding in Obsessive-Compulsive Disorder and Related Disorders: A Preliminary Report of 15 Cases." *Psychiatry and Clinical Neurosciences* 56: 17–23.

Stein, D. J. (2002). "Obsessive-Compulsive Disorder." *Lancet* 360: 397–406.

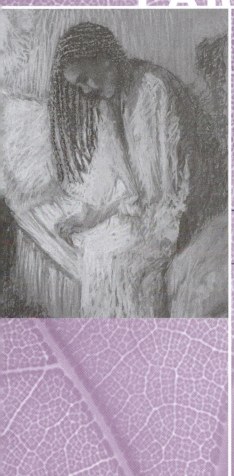

PART THREE

*The Client
Experiencing
Depression
or Mania*

Max

GENDER

M

AGE

12

SETTING

- Children's unit of a children and adolescent residential treatment center

ETHNICITY

- White American

CULTURAL CONSIDERATIONS

PREEXISTING CONDITION

COEXISTING CONDITION

COMMUNICATION

DISABILITY

SOCIOECONOMIC

- Single-parent home
- Mother works two jobs

SPIRITUAL/RELIGIOUS

PHARMACOLOGIC

PSYCHOSOCIAL

LEGAL

- Justification, doctor's order
- Documentation for room search

ETHICAL

- When is it ethical to search a child's room?

ALTERNATIVE THERAPY

PRIORITIZATION

DELEGATION

DEPRESSION OR MANIA

Level of difficulty: Moderate

Overview: Requires ability to assess for suicide ideation, answer various questions, and teach about depression. The nurse must set priorities around an order calling for this client to undergo "1:1 observation within eyesight at all times," and investigate the possibility of a suicide pact.

45

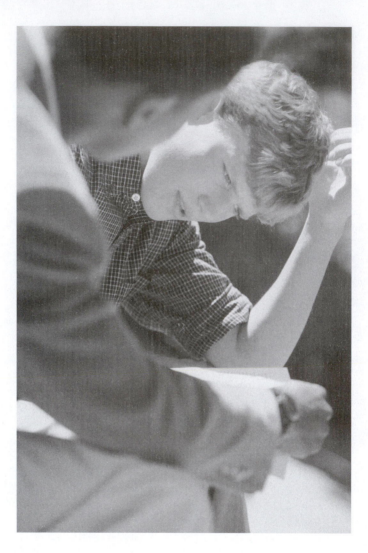

Client Profile

Max is a 12-year-old boy whose father died about five years ago. His father experienced periodic episodes of depression during his lifetime. After his father's death, Max displayed tantrums and became more aggressive toward his toys and people. He took on a serious, almost sad expression. He seemed empty and alone, even when in a room full of people. Max saw a therapist; after a period of play therapy, he stopped being more aggressive than boys his age, began to smile, and played with peers.

Max's mother went to work after his father's death; she now works two jobs. When she is home, she is authoritarian in her parenting style. Recently, Max's mother snooped around Max's room and found some morbid pictures that he had drawn (i.e., pictures of funerals, cemeteries, and people being shot or knifed to death). She also found cigarettes; as a consequence, he cannot have any friends visit and he may not leave the house except to go to school.

Max is not turning in schoolwork and is picking fights at school. In the evening, he plays video games and makes excuses for procrastinating with his homework. He lies awake at night worrying about his homework and things such as failing school, disappointing his mother, not having friends, and wondering if everyone hates him. When his mother tells him he is going to fail school, he responds, "I don't care."

The school nurse notices Max's behavior and becomes concerned, especially since two other students recently attempted suicide. She shares this information with Max's mother and suggests that a health care provider see Max. His mother takes him to a sliding-fee-scale clinic where a family practice health care provider who volunteers at the clinic sees Max. The health care provider identifies depression as a problem, considers putting Max on medication, but decides instead to have him admitted to a residential treatment center for evaluation and treatment. A clinic social worker finds funding from various sources to cover the cost of residential treatment at a facility for children and adolescents. The facility has child and adolescent psychiatrists and psychiatric nurses on staff.

Case Study

The nurse on the children's unit of the residential treatment center receives word Max will be admitted for treatment of depression. When Max and his mother arrive, the nurse does an intake interview with Max alone and then with both Max and his mother. Then the nurse interviews his mother while someone orients Max to the unit and its rules. Next, the nurse interviews Max alone while his mother tours the unit; she receives a copy of the parent handbook. Both Max and his mother are asked to sign a form indicating they have read the unit rules and will abide by them. Max's belongings are inventoried; some are locked up, while he is permitted to keep others. The child psychiatrist prescribes fluoxetine (Prozac) as well as individual and group therapy.

One night, Max gets irritable with the nurse for not letting him stay up past unit bedtime to watch his favorite television show. Max says, "It doesn't matter because I am just going to kill myself tonight anyway." The psychiatrist writes orders for Max to be placed on 1:1 observation within eyesight of an assigned staff member at all times. The following day Max learns he can't go to the recreation building because a unit rule states, "Anyone who threatens to kill himself or herself cannot leave the unit until he or she no longer wishes to kill himself or herself and twenty-four hours have past." Max tells the nurse, "I was just kidding. I really wasn't going to kill myself."

Questions

1. Why is Max being treated on a residential inpatient unit rather than on an outpatient basis?

2. On admission, would you ask Max directly if he is thinking about hurting himself or killing himself? What other questions would you ask?

3. Who should sign the informed consent form before Max takes fluoxetine? What teaching is needed about this medication prior to giving consent?

4. Max's mother tells you about the two other students who attempted suicide recently. How should you respond?

5. A new aide on the unit asks you, "What symptoms of depression are common in children and adolescents? Does Max have those symptoms?" What answers would you give?

6. What criteria would Max have to meet to warrant a diagnosis of Major Depressive Episode or Major Depressive Disorder? Could he possibly have Bipolar Disorder?

7. Max's mother asks you, "What causes depression in children or adolescents? Is it more common in males than in females? Is it hereditary?" How would you respond?

8. What is the incidence of depression in children and adolescents? Is it increasing or decreasing?

9. Max tells you about his mother's snooping, saying, "I think it is wrong for her to search my room. I hate her." What is your response?

10. To leave the unit, Max says, "I was just kidding. I really wasn't going to kill myself." How should you respond?

11. What data would you like to gather on Max prior to writing a nursing care plan?

12. What nursing diagnoses would you write for Max? What goals would you write? What interventions do you think would be helpful?

Questions and Suggested Answers

1. Why is Max being treated on a residential inpatient unit rather than on an outpatient basis? Several reasons justify admitting Max to a residential treatment center based on clinical judgment and concurrent parent report. His behavior indicates that he is depressed enough to consider killing or hurting himself. Especially troublesome, he is drawing pictures of cemeteries and funerals. Further, his mother works two jobs and can't watch him; even if she were home, she could not watch him twenty-four hours a day.

While the health care provider contemplates medication to treat Max's depression, recent warnings about selective serotonin reuptake inhibitors

(SSRIs) and increased suicide rates in children likely influenced deci-sion making. It could be that SSRIs lift the depression sufficiently to give the person enough energy to carry out his or her suicide plan. Nursing schools teach students to be especially vigilant when a client who is seri-ously depressed suddenly brightens, especially after being on medication or on other treatments because of increased energy levels. In addition, the health care provider might be concerned about who will follow up with Max if he prescribes on an outpatient basis. There is no guarantee that his mother will follow through with treatment or schedule outpatient follow-up. Likewise, if Max's suicidal threat is not taken seriously, the health care provider would be hard pressed to defend prescribing an SSRI, given the media frenzy about SSRIs and suicide.

In a facility with professional staff watching Max around the clock, he can safely start taking an SSRI. There, the child psychiatrist can adjust his medication as necessary. The facility also enables Max to deal with his issues in individual and group therapy and learn new ways to think and behave.

2. On admission, would you ask Max directly if he is thinking about hurt-ing himself or killing himself? What other questions would you ask? It is important to ask Max if he has thoughts about hurting or killing himself. Even though nurses know that a client can lie, lying about suicidal ideation is not common. If the client answers that he is thinking about killing him-self, then you need to determine whether he has devised a method for killing himself. If this answer is yes, then you need to ascertain whether he has access to this or any other method. The client with a method in mind and access to that method is considered at greater risk.

3. Who should sign the informed consent form before Max takes fluox-etine? What teaching is needed about this medication prior to giving consent? Max's mother should sign the informed consent form. In many facilities where children and adolescents receive psychotropic medications, adolescents also are asked to sign informed consent forms. There is no legal requirement for the minor to sign this form, however, the process makes the client more informed and increases the likelihood of complying with medication regimens.

Relative to teaching, you should alert Max and his mother to the fact that SSRIs can take four weeks or more to lessen depression. You should describe the possible side effects, including changes in appetite, insom-nia, increased anxiety, nausea, and agitation. You should underscore the importance of not abruptly stopping SSRI medications; they must be tapered under medical supervision. You should advise the mother that at least one recent study (Wohlfarth et al., 2004) found that SSRIs caused an increase in suicidal behavior, albeit a nonsignificant increase, in a group of children and adolescents taking SSRIs versus placebos. On the other hand, another group (Wong et al., 2004) reviewed current information on SSRIs and suicidality in children and adolescents (ideation, self-harm, and attempts) and found insufficient proof for an association between the two. Potts and Mandleco (2002) state, "SSRIs dominate the psychotherapy of depression because of their relatively safe side effect profile, very low lethality after overdose, and easy administration (once a day)."

4.   Max's mother tells you about the two other students who attempted suicide recently. How should you respond? You should encourage her to talk to the psychiatrist about this concern and facilitate a meeting between the two. Next, you should find out whether or not Max knows these students and if they have been in communication. Some students make suicide pacts wherein several students all agree to kill themselves. You need to probe to find out if Max was part of any such agreement. It could be that Max's school is so large that three suicidal students at one time can be due to the sheer size of the school or mere chance or coincidence.

5.   A new aide on the unit asks you, "What symptoms of depression are common in children and adolescents? Does Max have those symptoms?" What answers would you give? While adults tend to feel sad or empty, the mood of children and adolescents is somewhat irritable (APA, 2000). They can exhibit other symptoms, too. The *Harvard Mental Health Letter* (2002) describes the common symptoms of depression in children at various ages. Children younger than age three possess signs and symptoms that include "feeding problems, tantrums, and lack of playfulness and emotional expressiveness (Harvard Mental Health Letter, 1)." Between ages 3 and 5, depressed children might exhibit phobias and be accident-prone. Around age 5, children might engage in self-reproach exhibited in behavior such as "apologizing unnecessarily for minor mistakes and transgressions like spilling food or forgetting to put clothes away." From ages 6 to 8, children sometimes exhibit depression through verbalizing vague physical complaints and being aggressive. Some depressed children cling to parents and avoid new people and challenges. Between ages 9 and 12, children often show depression by lying awake worrying about schoolwork and other things, having morbid thoughts, and blaming themselves for disappointing their parents. Adolescents who are depressed might exhibit depression through angry behavior rather than sad. They might stop communicating and be hypersensitive to criticism. They can be annoying to parents and others. They also might exhibit depression through delinquent behavior such as running away, driving recklessly, stealing things, abusing alcohol and drugs, and expressing feelings of hopelessness.

Focus Adolescent Services (2005) presents these fifteen additional signs of depression in teens on its website:

1. Frequent sadness, tearfulness, and/or crying (wearing black clothes, writing morbid poetry, or playing music with nihilistic content can signify sadness)
2. Decreased interest in and ability to enjoy previously favorite activities (e.g., dropping out of sports, clubs, or activities)
3. Persistent boredom and low energy, sometimes manifested in a loss of concentration followed by lower grades or skipping school
4. Social isolation and poor communication
5. Low self-esteem and guilt
6. Extreme sensitivity to rejection or failure exemplified by the belief that they must reject family before family rejects them or by being critical, sarcastic, or abusive to others
7. Increased irritability, anger, or hostility
8. Difficulty with relationships
9. Physical complaints such as headache or stomachache
10. Frequently missing school
11. Poor concentration
12. Big changes in eating or sleeping habits
13. Threatening to run away or actually running away from home
14. Talking about suicide or self-injurious behavior
15. Abusing alcohol or other drugs and self-injurious behavior such as cutting or burning self

Temper tantrums and aggressiveness are common in children after the loss of a parent and in children who are depressed without loss as well. At the time of their appearance, Max was likely grieving the loss of his father, and these signs and symptoms expressed his unresolved grief. However, Max is now displaying somewhat different symptoms, ones that are common signs of depression in children his age. He is beyond the period for normal grieving, and he has a family history of depression. Thus, his symptoms appear to be a result of depression.

6. What criteria would Max have to meet to warrant a diagnosis of Major Depressive Episode or Major Depressive Disorder? Could he possibly have Bipolar Disorder? To be diagnosed with Major Depressive Disorder, Recurrent, Max would need to have had two or more Major Depressive Episodes (described below) that cannot be accounted for by thought disorders (e.g., Schizophrenia). Further, he could not have ever had a manic episode, a mixed episode (mania and depression in one episode), or a hypomanic-like episode. According to the *Diagnostic and Statistical Manual of Mental Disorders* (APA, 2000, 376), "To be considered separate Major Depressive

Disorder episodes, there must be an interval of at least two consecutive months in which criteria are not met for a Major Depressive Disorder."

Max could be diagnosed as having a Major Depressive Episode if he meets five of the following nine criteria:

1. Depressed or irritable mood nearly every day for most of the day (more often irritable in children but could be depressed)
2. A greatly diminished or absent interest or pleasure in things that were previously interesting or pleasurable mostly all day every day (i.e., anhedonia)
3. Failure to make expected weight gains
4. Not sleeping enough or sleeping too much
5. Psychomotor agitation or retardation nearly every day
6. Fatigue or loss of energy almost every day
7. Excessive or inappropriate guilt or feelings of worthlessness nearly every day
8. Reduced ability to concentrate, make decisions, or think nearly every day (can be self-reported or observed by others)
9. Recurrent thoughts of death and recurrent suicide ideation that can involve a specific plan or a suicide attempt or not

These symptoms must not be attributable to medical conditions or substance abuse, or better-accounted-for by grieving the loss of a loved one. The symptoms also must cause clinically significant distress in important areas of the child's life such as school or socialization.

The possibility exists that this client will, sometime later in his life, have a manic episode and be diagnosed as having Bipolar Disorder.

7. Max's mother asks you, "What causes depression in children or adolescents? Is it more common in males than in females? Is it hereditary?" How would you respond? It is probable that a number of complex factors are involved in causing depression. Lewis (2003) relates that health care providers and researchers think, "Depression may have a number of complex and interacting causes." Genetic research points to genetic differences that make a person vulnerable to depression. A hereditary component probably increases the risk of vulnerability to depression. Research also suggests a hereditary component, as the risk of vulnerability is greater if another person in the family manifests the same problem. It is likely that the genetic vulnerability is accompanied by strengths and risk factors. When the risk factors act in sufficient force to overcome the strengths, depression occurs. Risk factors include loss, trauma, hormonal changes, and physical and sexual abuse. Strengths include a supportive nurturing family, financial security, good looks, and charisma.

In prepubertal children such as Max, Major Depressive Disorder, whether a single episode or recurrent, affects girls and boys equally. In adolescence and adulthood, the disorder is twice as common in women as it is in men. The *Diagnostic and Statistical Manual of Mental Disorders* (APA, 2000, 373) states, "Major Depressive Disorder is 1.5–3 times more common among first-degree biological relatives of persons with this disorder than among the general population."

Dysthymic Disorder is a chronically depressed mood occurring almost every day, more days than not, for at least one year in children and adolescents and two years in adults. It is said to occur equally in both sexes in children, and two to three times more often in women than in men. It is more common among first-degree biologic relatives of those with Dysthymic Disorder (APA, 2000).

8. What is the incidence of Depression in children and adolescents? Is it increasing or decreasing? From estimates of the incidence of Major Depressive Disorder, figures on the percentage of childhood sufferers at various ages are: 1 percent in preschoolers, 2 percent in children from ages 6 through 12, and 5–9 percent in early to late adolescence. Dysthymic Disorder occurs at a rate of about 0.6–1.7 percent in children and 1.6–8 percent in adolescents. The *Harvard Mental Health Letter* (2002, 1) states, "More than 2/3rds of children with dysthymia develop major depression within five years."

Health care providers are recognizing depressive disorders at earlier ages than in the past, and, since 1940, their incidence has increased with each new generation.

9. Max tells you about his mother's snooping, saying, "I think it is wrong for her to search my room. I hate her." What is your response? Using reflection, a therapeutic communication tool, you could say, "I hear you saying that your mother's behavior upset you." This statement gives Max the chance to identify and ventilate his feelings about his mother's behavior and to begin to recognize that he hates his mother's behavior but does not hate his mother. After he responds, you could even say, "It sounds to me that you don't really hate your mother, you just hate what she did." You also could ask Max if he has any ideas on how to get his mother to trust him and stop snooping in his room. The focus should be on what behavioral changes Max could make to gain his mother's confidence. You might have him role play a parent and you (or a peer) could role play a child like Max. In the role play, he might discover a rationale for searching a child's room and, as the parent; he might be harsher on the child than his own mother.

"Snooping" parent behavior could be a topic for group discussion. Girls often discover their mothers have been reading their journals, diaries, or e-mails. Max will find he is not the only child in group therapy who has had a parent go through their belongings secretly. You also can raise this issue at the treatment team planning sessions. In both group and treatment team meetings, policies on searching a child's room or personal belongings need to be discussed.

Most facilities require an initial inventory of clients' belongings on admission, with certain items locked up during the hospital stay or used only under staff supervision. Once the client is admitted, most facilities require staff to get an order from the health care provider before searching a child's room. Any new items must be inventoried, with those not permitted on the unit locked up.

10. To leave the unit, Max says, "I was just kidding. I really wasn't going to kill myself." How should you respond? You need to explain to Max the seriousness of his threat, saying, "We take every threat to hurt yourself or kill yourself very seriously here. You might think you are kidding, but whether you are or not doesn't matter. We must take it seriously." Then, you should cite the unit rule that requires him to remain on the unit. Some units give the nurse the option of allowing a suicidal client to go off the unit with an escort. In that case, you could assign an escort and let Max go to the gym. Many nurses and staff feel strongly that clients who threaten suicide should have tightened security, thereby learning that there are consequences for being viewed as suicidal, whether the client is joking or not. The nurse must know the facility's policies about suicidal clients being allowed off the unit as well as the rules governing observation of suicidal clients.

11. What data would you like to gather on Max prior to writing a nursing care plan? You need to obtain the client's weight and height for a baseline. You should ask Max about his appetite and then observe him during mealtimes to learn how depression is affecting his appetite and his weight. You need to observe his sleep patterns as charted and discuss them with Max, his mother, and other staff. You must ask Max about his nicotine use and any drug or alcohol use. You also should ask about his interests and hobbies.

Reading the history and physical done by the health care provider on admission might reveal that a drug screen was performed. Together, an examination and drug screen can rule out medical disorders or drugs that can cause depression (e.g., hypo- and hyperthyroidism, Addison's disease, drug abuse, and withdrawal). The examination also will detect any injuries, accidental or otherwise. Documentation of skin condition on admission will facilitate identification of new injuries that are self-inflicted or due to neglect or abuse by staff. Depression rating scales and self-report instruments such as the Children's Depression Inventory, the Beck Depression Inventory, and the Zung Self Rating Depression Scale are helpful too.

12. What nursing diagnoses would you write for Max? What goals would you write? What interventions do you think would be helpful? Nursing diagnoses include risk for self-directed violence, self-esteem chronic low; social interaction impaired; social isolation; and sleep pattern disturbed. Possible goals for this client are

- Will state positive affirmations during each waking shift
- Will sleep eight to ten hours each night
- Will engage in 90 percent of classes and other unit activities
- Will have no instances of self-harm

Helpful interventions include

- Applying rules consistently
- Encouraging client to attend all scheduled therapy

Cognitive Behavioral Therapy (CBT) with or without parental involvement is effective in treating childhood depression (Fonagy and Target, 2003). The nursing care plan also can include interventions by staff nurses that support CBT, such as teaching the client about "thinking errors" and how to identify and stop these thinking errors and substitute problem-solving behaviors or other healthy behaviors. Clients can be encouraged to do positive affirmations as well.

Group therapy might be especially helpful due to the strength of peer influence in adolescent clients. One example is the power of the group when confronting someone exhibiting a thinking error. The group can be supportive as well as gently confrontational.

A nurse can be assigned to be Max's primary nurse for the length of his stay or at least to have 1:1 interactions with the client on a regular basis. An important intervention would be to develop a trusting therapeutic relationship with Max and with his mother.

The admitting or treating psychiatrist might order family therapy. Wang and Crane (2001) identify specific family transactional characteristics in children with physiologic vulnerability to psychosomatic illness. The four transactional characteristics are enmeshment, overprotectiveness, rigidity, and lack of conflict resolution. In family therapy, the therapist will look at how Max and his mother interact and help them find healthy ways to interact.

In addition to teaching the mother and client about the SSRI prescribed, interventions include being alert for side effects, asking the client to open his mouth after taking the pills, and checking for any cheeking of medication. Wong and associates (2004) state, "SSRIs should not be considered for use as front line treatment in mild or moderate depression of childhood, where psychological interventions such as cognitive behavior therapy or interpersonal therapy are the mainstay." They believe that SSRIs should be reserved for the child who is suicidal and/or has severe depression and is admitted to an inpatient unit. Nurses working with children who are depressed will find that some prescribing health care providers have a different view of when SSRIs are to be used with children.

Except for nurse practitioners, the nurse does not decide whether clients receive medication or what medication they take. However, the nurse must keep informed on medications for depression in childhood and adolescence by keeping up with the literature and discussing clients' medication with the prescribing health care provider.

References

American Psychiatric Association (APA). (2000). *Diagnostic and Statistical Manual of Mental Disorders, 4th ed.* Text Revision. Washington, DC: APA.

"Depression in Children—Part I." (2002). *Harvard Mental Health Letter* 18(8): 1–4.

Focus Adolescent Services. "Teen Depression: Warning Signs, Information, Getting Help." www.focusas.com/Depression.html. Accessed December 1, 2005.

Fonagy, P. and M. Target. (2003). "A Review of Outcomes of MH Interventions for Children and Adolescents." *The Brown University Child and Adolescent Behavior Letter* (February): 1, 6–7.

Lewis, C. (2003). "The Lowdown on Depression." *FDA Consumer* 37(1): 28–34.

Potts, N. L. and B. Mandleco. (2002). *Pediatric Nursing: Caring for Children and Their Families.* Clifton Park, NJ: Thomson Delmar Learning.

Wohlfarth, T., et al. (2004). "Use of Serotonin Reuptake Inhibitors in Childhood Depression." *Lancet* 364(9435): 659–660.

Wang, L. and D. R. Crane. (2001). "The Relationship Between Marital Satisfaction, Marital Stability, Nuclear Family Triangulation, and Childhood Depression." *American Journal of Family Therapy* 29: 337–347.

Wong, I. C., et al. (2004). "Use of Selective Serotonin Reuptake Inhibitors in Children and Adolescents." *Drug Safety* 27(13): 991–1000.

Emily

GENDER

F

AGE

22

SETTING

- Community mental health center

ETHNICITY

- White American

CULTURAL CONSIDERATIONS

- Working university student

PREEXISTING CONDITION

COEXISTING CONDITION

COMMUNICATION

DISABILITY

SOCIOECONOMIC

SPIRITUAL/RELIGIOUS

PHARMACOLOGIC

- Lamotrigine (Lamictal)

PSYCHOSOCIAL

LEGAL

ETHICAL

- Should client withhold information or lie to get her insurance application accepted?

ALTERNATIVE THERAPY

- St. John's wort

PRIORITIZATION

DELEGATION

MODERATE

BIPOLAR II

Level of difficulty: Moderate

Overview: Requires use of therapeutic communication, observation, and listening skills to elicit symptoms and other information that the psychiatrist can use to arrive at an accurate diagnosis.

Client Profile

Emily is a 22-year-old female whose mother died in a car accident when she was age 5. After her mother's death, Emily became irritable, impulsive, and hyperactive at times; refused to eat; and looked sad. Her father took her to a child psychiatrist who believed she was depressed over the loss of her mother and treated her for situational depression. He noted that Emily's maternal grandfather had been admitted to the state hospital with depression. The grandfather, who ran a large business, did well between episodes of depression.

About a year after her mother's death, Emily's mood seemed to improve, but she struggled in school with irritability, distractibility, impulsivity, and periodic depressed moods. Her teachers wondered if she had Attention Deficit Hyperactivity Disorder. During adolescence, she saw both a psychiatrist and a therapist for depression. Her father kept a file detailing her visits to mental health professionals, and Emily received the file when she was 18 years old.

After high-school graduation, Emily feared she would not do well in college, so she began working as a waitress. At age 22, she enrolled in a community college part time. Her plan was to take classes in the morning, work in the afternoon and evening, and study at night because she was experiencing more energy than she had in the past. For a few days she had more energy at night and required only three or four hours of sleep. She felt more goal-directed. Then the depressed mood returned. She experienced three or four Major Depressive Episodes and at least two periods of increased energy which Emily thinks of as normal, but may be Hypomanic Episodes, in the past twelve months. Emily is now feeling depressed and unable to focus on school.

Case Study

Emily keeps her first appointment at the community mental health center. She has no medical or mental health insurance coverage. She wants a psychiatrist to prescribe medication to stop the depressive episodes and help her concentrate better. A nurse introduces herself and tells Emily they will talk before she sees the health care provider. Emily hands the nurse the file containing her past mental health assessments and treatments saying, "This file probably explains it all." The nurse tells Emily they need to chat regardless. During the nurse's assessment, Emily shares that her energy is down, she feels fatigued, feels worthless at times, and can't concentrate, but that her energy goes up sometimes like two weeks ago when it was up and she suddenly had all kinds of neat ideas, wanted to talk to people, accomplish things, and even her libido was increased and she wanted to date again. Emily also describes a recent shopping spree in which she bought pans, dishes, silverware, glassware, small appliances, and other things using her credit card. Later, a friend convinced her to take everything back since she could not afford the purchases.

The nurse does a thorough assessment on Emily and documents her findings for the psychiatrist. He uses this information, as well as his own assessment findings and Emily's file, to diagnose her as having Bipolar II Disorder. He believes she is rapid cycling, writes a prescription for lamotrigine (Lamictal); he indicates he might later add a selective serotonin reuptake inhibitor (SSRI) such as sertraline (Zoloft). He asks the nurse to do some medication teaching with the client.

Emily returns to the community mental health center two weeks later for a follow-up evaluation. She tells the nurse she applied for health insurance but her application was denied because of the Bipolar II diagnosis. She asks the nurse, "Should I try another insurance company and lie on the insurance form?"

Questions

1. How would you respond to Emily's statement that her file "says it all"? Give your rationale.

2. What would help you get a clearer picture of this client's moods? What other questions would you ask? What observations would be important to the psychiatrist (in diagnosing) and the team (in treatment planning)?

3. Since the client only mentions depression, why is it important to know about the client's variations in mood, especially manic moods and moods falling between normal and manic? What is a Mixed Episode (in a person with Bipolar I)?

4. What are the criteria for a diagnosis of Bipolar II Disorder?

5. What are the similarities and differences in criteria for a Manic Episode and a Hypomanic Episode? Looking at the symptoms of Manic Episodes and Hypomanic Episodes, how would you assess this client for these signs, especially for inflated self-esteem or grandiosity?

6. Is the shopping spree Emily described a manic rather than a hypomanic behavior? Give examples of hypomanic and manic behavior.

7. The client asks, "Why isn't the health care provider adding sertraline now?" What do you think is the reason?

8. You must teach the client about lamotrigine (Lamictal). What would you include in your teaching? Emily asks you about taking St. John's wort for depression. What is your response?

9. The client asks, "What did the health care provider mean by rapid cycling?" What is your response?

10. The client asks, "Do people with Bipolar II have less depression and less time ill than people with Bipolar I?" What is your answer?

11. What is the cause of Bipolar II? What is the usual age of onset? What is the incidence?

12. What nursing diagnoses and goals would you write for this client? What interventions would be most helpful?

13. How should you respond to Emily's question regarding lying on an insurance form?

Questions and Suggested Answers

1. How would you respond to Emily's statement that her file "says it all"? Give your rationale. One option is to say, "Tell me in your own words what is going on with you." Another states, "You are the expert Emily. I want to hear about you, from you." You might have a different but equally good response. Regardless of approach, the client must provide you a clear, first-hand report of moods, thoughts, and behaviors. You must update the information others have gathered, adding to it and correcting erroneous data. Even if the client comes without a file, these statements are good for opening the initial interview.

2. What would help you get a clearer picture of this client's moods? What other questions would you ask? What observations would be important to the psychiatrist (in diagnosing) and the team (in treatment planning)? To get a better idea of the client's mood changes during her waking hours, you can ask her to graph her moods over the past twenty-four hours. A convenient scale is: 0 = the most depressed state imaginable; 5 = normal; and 10 = manic or very energetic. The client can continue graphing her mood changes daily for the next few weeks and bring these graphs to her next appointment. Then, you can ask the client any of the following questions:

- What do you feel like when you are most depressed? What do you do?
- What is the most energetic you get?
- What is something you do when you are at your most energetic?
- How much of the day do you feel irritated? What seems to trigger your irritation?

Antai-Otong (2004) suggests asking the following questions to identify whether or not the client has had episodes of hypomania:

- Have you ever had a time in your life when you had a lot of energy, did not need a lot of sleep, and felt creative?
- How much sleep do you get at night? Are there nights when you get less sleep? How much less? What causes this, and what do you do when you don't sleep?
- What medicines are you currently taking? What medicines have you taken in the past?
- Are you allergic to any medicines, or have you had any adverse or unusual reactions to medications?
- Has anyone in your family ever had a mood disorder such as Dysthymia, Depression, Bipolar I, or Bipolar II?
- Do you know the mental health histories of relatives on both sides of your family? If not, is there a relative you can ask?

You should observe the client's manner of dress. Depressed clients usually select somber clothing that is darker in color and more conservative. The person with hypomania might select a few bright colors or accessories and will tend not to be conservative in the choice of clothing. The female client with mania, who often is hypersexual, might select more colorful, somewhat flamboyant clothing and/or clothing that is tight, short, and low cut.

You also should observe the client's affect (i.e., emotional response to what is said or what the client is experiencing). As you watch both the client's face and body reactions, you might notice that sometimes the client's response is "blunted" or greatly diminished compared to the average person. In other cases, the client's response is "flat" (i.e., the facial muscles don't move and there is little or no reaction). The client's reaction also could be characterized as "labile" if she's rapidly moving from one affect to another (e.g., from animated to blunted). You can determine whether or not the affect is appropriate (i.e., when discussing something that is tragic or sad, the client has a sad expression and is not giggling).

You also should observe the client's behavior (e.g., sitting still or pacing). On occasion, you will see some odd or puzzling behaviors. You need to describe them as objectively as possible in your charting. Observation is a powerful assessment tool.

3. Since the client only mentions depression, why is it important to know about the client's variations in mood, especially manic moods and moods falling between normal and manic? What is a Mixed Episode (in a person with Bipolar I)? A person diagnosed with Major Depressive Disorder could eventually have that diagnosis changed to Bipolar I or Bipolar II. You must look for clues in mood and behavior that will help the psychiatrist rule out or select a diagnosis from the various mood disorder diagnoses. It is especially important for clients who might have Bipolar II. Some recognize only their depressed moods and might think their hypomanic moods are normal.

The most important criteria a client has to meet to be diagnosed as having Bipolar I Disorder is the occurrence of at least one Manic Episode in the past or a Mixed Episode. Interestingly, a client can be diagnosed as having Bipolar I Disorder, Single Manic Episode without ever having a Major Depressive Episode. This apparently assumes a Major Depressive Episode will occur in the future since *bipolar* implies two poles of mood. If the person has had a Depressive Episode in the past and experiences a Manic Episode, then the diagnosis becomes Bipolar I Disorder.

To qualify for a diagnosis of Mixed Episode, the client must have both a manic episode and a Major Depressive Episode during the same period of time. It must last for at least one week. The client must exhibit rapidly alternating moods, along with symptoms of mania and Major Depressive

Disorder, occurring nearly every day for one week or more; these symptoms must be severe enough to cause impairment in functioning in some area of the person's life or require hospitalization to prevent any harm to the client or others, or the client must have psychotic features.

4. What are the criteria for a diagnosis of Bipolar II? In order to be diagnosed with Bipolar II Disorder, the client must:

- Present with or have a history of at least one Major Depressive Episodes
- Present with or have history of one or more Hypomanic Episodes
- Never have suffered a Manic Episode or a Mixed Episode
- Experience clinically significant distress from the symptoms or impairment in some important area of functioning such as social and/or occupational (work or school)

The depressive and hypomanic symptoms must not be better accounted for by another psychiatric or medical disorder from the Schizoaffective Disorders or must not be added onto Schizophrenia, Schiophreniform Disorder, Delusional Disorder, or Psychotic Disorder Not Otherwise Specified. Also, they must not be accounted for by a medical diagnosis or result from medication or abuse of a substance (APA, 2000).

5. What are the similarities and differences in criteria for a Manic Episode and a Hypomanic Episode? Looking at the symptoms of Manic Episodes and Hypomanic Episodes, how would you assess this client for these signs, especially for inflated self-esteem or grandiosity? According to the *Diagnostic and Statistical Manual of Mental Disorders* (APA, 2000), the seven criteria (signs) are exactly the same for a Manic Episode or a Hypomanic Episode:

1. Having inflated self-esteem or sense of grandiosity
2. Requiring less sleep
3. Talking more than usual
4. Moving from one idea to another or feeling as if thoughts are racing
5. Being easily distracted by external stimuli
6. Experiencing more goal-directed activity than usual or psychomotor agitation
7. Pursuing pleasurable activities excessively with a high risk for painful consequences (e.g., buying sprees, sexual involvement, or unwise business investing)

For a Manic Episode, a person must have a distant period of "abnormally and persistently elevated, expansive, or irritable mood," lasting at least one week (or any duration if hospitalization is necessary), (APA, 2000, 357) and three of the seven symptoms to a significant degree, or four if the mood is only irritable. The criteria for a Hypomanic Episode omits the word "abnormally" from the quote above. The Hypomanic Episode must last at least four days. The criteria for number of symptoms are the same for both Manic Episode and Hypomanic Episode. The differences between the two lie in the degree of impairment in the client's life, whether hospitalization is needed, and whether there is psychosis. The Manic Episode criteria require that the mood disturbance be severe enough to cause marked impairment in important aspects of the person's life or require hospitalization to reduce risk of harm to self and others or exhibit psychotic features. The Hypomanic Episode requires that the episode *not be severe enough* to cause impairment in significant areas of the person's life or cause hospitalization or exhibit psychotic features. The criteria for Hypomanic Episode also require that the changes in functioning and the disturbance in mood be observable to others and be a change in functioning uncharacteristic of the person when asymptomatic.

There are a number of ways to measure self-esteem and determine whether grandiosity exists. One simple way is to listen to themes in what the person is saying. Is the client humble or do you hear a theme of bragging on self? Is the person portraying herself, or her family, as being better, more important, or more intelligent or possessing more money or having done something spectacular? You could ask the client what she says to herself when she looks in the mirror, or how she would describe herself to others. You can ask her to describe the accomplishment of which she is most proud.

You have already assessed for amount of sleep required. Assessing for being more talkative than usual, racing ideas/thoughts, and being more easily distracted than usual can be done by listening and simply asking if the person sometimes feels pressured to talk or if her thoughts seem to be racing at times or if she has difficulty concentrating on one thing at a time.

Excessive pursuit of pleasure might be hard to elicit, but you might try asking the client if she has had any fun or unusual experiences lately.

6. Is the shopping spree Emily described a manic rather than a hypomanic behavior? Give examples of hypomanic and manic behavior. An example of a shopping spree by a client with hypomanic behaviors is buying a lot of things in a short period of time, but probably returning them later. Manic persons might go on a shopping spree, but will buy things for which they have no use (e.g., a set of expensive drums when they don't play drums), and they might give items away to someone they don't even know. A hypomanic person might be more sexual than usual, but a manic person might be dancing nude on the table in a bar or openly propositioning the staff and others for sex.

7.   The client asks, "Why isn't the health care provider adding sertraline now?" What do you think is the reason? There is a possibility that SSRI antidepressants taken initially as a single drug therapy without mood stabilizers can precipitate manic or hypomanic episodes. Hadjipavlou and associates (2004) suggest that the problem of SSRIs causing mood switching may not be as prevalent as previously thought, but are still cautious and advise starting a client with Bipolar II on a trial of either Lithium or lamotrigine as first-line drugs. According to Hadjipavlou and associates (2004), if this works, it should be continued on a long-term basis; if it does not achieve good results, then an antidepressant should be added to the mood stabilizer.

If the physician eventually prescribes sertraline and Emily cannot afford to buy it, she can check with the drug companies producing SSRIs. These companies advertise that they have programs to assist people who need these drugs and cannot afford them.

8.   You must teach the client about lamotrigine. What would you include in your teaching? Emily asks you about taking St. John's wort for depression. What is your response? You can tell the client that lamotrigine is an anticonvulsant that also is effective as a mood stabilizer in rapid-cycling Bipolar II Disorder. You would tell the client about the side effects and instruct her to withhold the drug and report any rashes immediately. Some serious rashes have been reported after lamotrigine use that required hospitalization, especially in children. Antai-Otong (2004, 126) points out that "a major drawback of lamotrigine (Lamictal) is its side effect profile that requires slow titration to reduce the risk of severe rash.... Another concern with the use of this medication as monotherapy is its failure to protect against relapse or breakthrough depression."

Clients report a wide variety of side effects, so Emily should be told to report any new symptoms that might be associated with the drug. Periodic complete blood cell (CBC) counts need to be done, as hematologic side effects have occurred in a small number of cases.

A number of medications lower lamotrigine levels including acetaminophen, carbamazepine, oral contraceptives, and phenobarbital; valproic acid and other drugs increase lamotrigine levels. Thus, the prescribing physician should be made aware of other drugs the client is taking.

The National Institute of Mental Health (NIMH; 2001) advises persons thinking about trying herbal or natural supplements to discuss it first with their doctor, indicating that findings suggest that medication effectiveness can be lessened by concurrent use of St. John's wort. NIMH also suggests that persons with bipolar disorder who are not on a mood stabilizer can experience mania or hypomania after taking St. John's wort.

9.   The client asks, "What did the health care provider mean by rapid cycling?" What is your response? The term *rapid cycling* is used with Bipolar I or Bipolar II. It simply means that the client experienced four or more mood episodes in the previous twelve-month period. The mood episodes can be Manic, Hypomanic, or Mixed Episodes, but there must be full remission between episodes, or there must be a switch to an opposite polarity of mood. All episodes must meet duration and symptom criteria for the episode type. Interestingly, 70–90 percent of people who are rapid cycling are female. Further, Bipolar II Disorder is thought to occur more frequently in females than males. Notably, Bipolar I is believed to occur equally in males and females (APA, 2000).

10. The client asks, "Do people with Bipolar II have less depression and less time ill than people with Bipolar I?" What is your answer? You should point out that everyone is different; thus, some people might experience deeper depression or longer periods of time ill, while others will not. You should mention that compliance with treatment could be a key factor in shorter periods of illness. Joffe and associates (2004) found that in both bipolar types the subjects spent half of their time in a so-called "normal" or euthymic mood with the balance spent in "varying severity of mood states." These researchers characterized subjects as mostly having "minor and subsyndromal symptoms," with no difference in the amount of time spent with depressive symptoms. Benazzi (2001) found that three out of four subjects with Bipolar Disorder II had increased levels of functioning in the hypomanic state; the remaining subject had only slight impairment.

11. What is the cause of Bipolar II? What is the usual age of onset? What is the incidence? The cause of Bipolar II Disorder is unknown, but likely has both a biochemical basis and a genetic component, as Bipolar II tends to run in families. Several genes might be involved, and the genetic component likely predisposes the person to Bipolar II rather than causes it.

Benazzi (2001) described early onset from ages 20–30 and late onset after age 30. Hadjipavlou and coworkers (2004, 809) state, "Bipolar II Disorder may be more common than previously thought; systematic probing improves early identification of the disorder." They suggest its incidence approaches 5 percent of the population.

12. What nursing diagnoses and goals would you write for this client? What interventions would be most helpful? Likely nursing diagnoses include disturbed sleep pattern; disturbed thought processes related to inability to concentrate, distractibility and racing thoughts; and knowledge deficit: symptom management and medication.

Appropriate goals include:

- Report an increase in sleep to five hours/twenty-four-hour period
- Report success in focusing on tasks

- Describe appropriate methods for dealing with symptoms
- Identify and use a system for remembering to take medication

Helpful interventions include:

- Having the client attend a group for clients with mood disorders to get support and share ideas about how to deal with symptoms, medication, and other concerns associated with mood disorders
- Having client think of ways to remember medication and reasons to comply with medication regimen
- Educating client about symptom management and medication, and assessing the client's understanding of this information
- Discussing various methods for remembering to take medication (e.g., pill boxes for each day of the week, calendars with names of medications to cross off each day, envelopes with medications for each day or each scheduled pill time)
- Talking with the client about recognizing racing thoughts and doing quiet activities alone to slow the thoughts

13. How should you respond to Emily's question regarding lying on an insurance form? Clients with bipolar or other psychiatric diagnoses commonly ask whether they should lie or omit information on insurance forms or job applications. This practice can prove problematic when the truth eventually comes out.

One of the best responses asks, "Do you have any other ideas of how to deal with this problem without lying?" In most cases, it is better to help the client follow a problem-solving process than providing a "fix-it" answer.

If you need to make suggestions, you might ask other people with a bipolar diagnosis how they solved this problem. You also could see what type of insurance the college offers and if it covers a psychiatric diagnosis. The local or state mental health association might be a good source of help.

References

American Psychiatric Association (APA). (2000). *Diagnostic and Statistical Manual of Mental Disorders, 4th ed.* Text Revision. Washington, DC: APA.

Antai-Otong, D. (2004). "Bipolar II or Unipolar Depression: Pharmacologic Considerations." *Perspectives in Psychiatric Care* 40(3):125–128.

Benazzi, F. (2001). "Early Onset Versus Late Onset Bipolar II Disorder." *Journal of Psychiatry and Nueroscience* 25(1): 53–57.

Hadjipavlou, G., et al. (2004). "Bipolar II Disorder: An Overview of Recent Developments." *Canadian Journal of Psychiatry* 49(12): 802–811.

Joffe, R. T., et al. (2004). "A Prospective, Longitudinal Study of Percentage of Time Spent Ill in Patients with Bipolar I or Bipolar II Disorders." *Bipolar Disorders* 6: 62–66.

National Institute of Mental Health (NIMH). (2001). *Bipolar Disorder.* Bethesda, MD: NIMH, National Institutes of Health. Available online at http://nimh.nih.gov/publicat/bipolar.cfm.

Parker, G. (2004). "Highlighting Bipolar II Disorder." *Canadian Journal of Psychiatry* 49(12): 791–793.

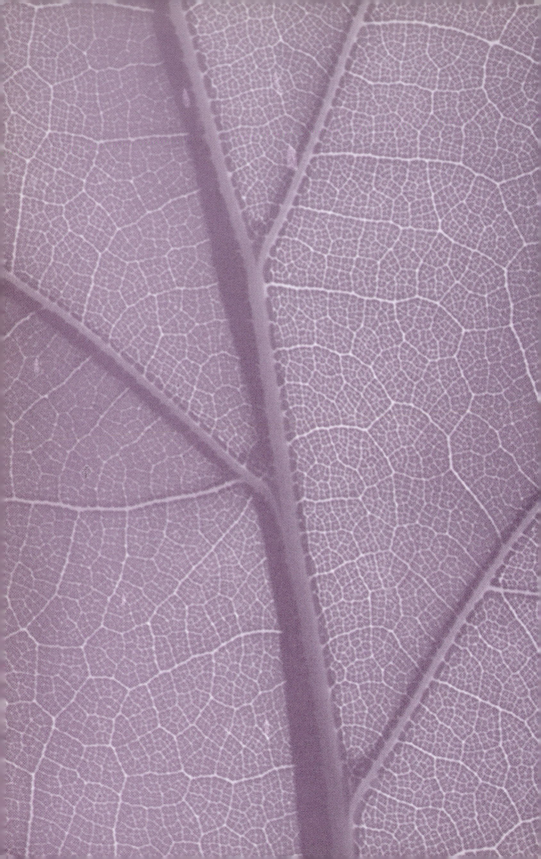

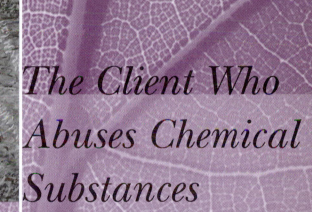

PART FOUR

The Client Who Abuses Chemical Substances

CASE STUDY 1

Jeff

GENDER

M

AGE

43

SETTING

- Inpatient treatment center for substance abuse and alcoholism

ETHNICITY

- White American

CULTURAL CONSIDERATIONS

- Small town

PREEXISTING CONDITION

- Attention Deficit Hyperactivity Disorder (ADHD)
- Traits of Conduct Disorder

COEXISTING CONDITION

- Gastritis
- Pancreatitis
- Nicotine addiction

COMMUNICATION

DISABILITY

SOCIOECONOMIC

- Loss of job
- Wife threatening to leave

SPIRITUAL/RELIGIOUS

- Atheist

PHARMACOLOGIC

- Chlordiazepoxide (Librium)
- Lorazepam (Ativan)
- Thiamine (vitamin B$_1$)

PSYCHOSOCIAL

- Socialization centered on drinking alcohol; avoids social events and people who do not drink alcohol

LEGAL

- Driving while intoxicated (DWI) charge
- Question of whether it is legal or not to require an atheist to attend Alcoholics Anonymous (AA) as part of court decision

ETHICAL

- Is it ethical for a private treatment program to require an atheist to attend AA and work on turning things over to God as part of the 12-step program?

ALTERNATIVE THERAPY

- Acupuncture
- Alpha stimulation

PRIORITIZATION

DELEGATION

MODERATE

CHEMICAL OR SUBSTANCE ABUSE

Level of difficulty: Moderate

Overview: Requires patience, understanding, and the ability to be empathic, therapeutic, and professional with a client who has abused alcohol to the point of compromising his health, placing others in danger, and hurting others. The nurse must be able to set firm limits and avoid manipulation; confront the client about denial issues; be supportive; and develop a trusting therapeutic relationship. The nurse must recognize the implications of the preexisting ADHD condition on instructions to the client.

71

Client Profile

Jeff is a 43-year-old white male who began drinking at age 12. His father kept alcohol in the home and Jeff secretively helped himself to it. He then began skipping school to drink with friends and his grades fell. The police picked him up for underage drinking when he was 17. His mother, who came to get him from jail, had bailed Jeff's grandfather out of jail many times for drunkenness and fighting in bars. Several other relatives were alcoholics. Jeff's mother took him to see a professional counselor who diagnosed Jeff as having Attention Deficit Disorder with Hyperactivity (ADHD) and Conduct Disorder traits, including problems with authority figures and breaking rules. The therapist told her, "Counseling would be a waste of money."

After high school, Jeff took a job in sales and drank at night with his coworkers. The amount he drank steadily increased. He married, but his wife divorced him and refused to let their two children ride in the car with him. Jeff remarried and continued his drinking. He began meeting some drinking buddies at the bowling alley. He would arrive before his friends and start drinking vodka on the rocks, his drink of choice. After a night of drinking, he would drive home and fall asleep in his car in the driveway, too drunk to go inside. Jeff often took oranges filled with vodka (via a syringe) to work. He needed the alcohol to keep from having the "shakes." Four Mondays in a row Jeff's wife called his employer to report Jeff being sick. His boss finally fired Jeff.

Jeff began to complain of stomach pain; he was diagnosed with gastritis and later pancreatitis. The doctor advised him to stop drinking any alcoholic beverages, but Jeff continued to drink. Jeff smokes nearly two packs of cigarettes a day. His children have unsuccessfully begged him to stop.

In Jeff's small town, there are only two places to socialize: bars and churches. Jeff claims he is atheist, so he hangs out in bars. Usually the town police overlook his weaving on the way home, but one night the state police pulled him over and charged him with driving while intoxicated (DWI). It was Jeff's second DWI in five years. His wife threatens to leave him if he does not go into treatment. Jeff's lawyer suggests an inpatient alcohol and drug treatment center, indicating things will go better for him in court if he is in treatment.

Case Study

Jeff presents to an inpatient alcohol and drug treatment center. His wife tells the nurse that Jeff drank a fifth of vodka the night before. When the nurse later asks Jeff about his alcohol use, he denies having a drinking problem. He indicates he is entering treatment to appease his wife and lawyer. The nurse asks Jeff when he had his last drink. Jeff truthfully responds that it was last night.

The health care provider writes orders for lorazepam (Ativan) 0.5–1 mg three times a day and every four hours as needed for agitation; chlordiazepoxide (Librium) 50 mg every six hours for four doses, then 25 mg every six hours for eight doses; a multiple vitamin; and thiamine. He also orders vital signs every four hours and instructs the client to attend a class on the effects of alcohol on the body; an in-house Alcoholics Anonymous (AA) group; recreational therapy; and individual, family, and group therapy.

On the second day of hospitalization, Jeff talks about his alcohol abuse in group therapy, saying how it has affected his life. He tells the group how he would weave while driving home from bars, but the police would let him go because it was a small town and he knew most of the force from high school. He described sleeping in the driveway every night because he was too drunk to walk into the house.

On day seven of his hospitalization, Jeff tells the group that he is going to leave treatment because he misses his wife and wants to sleep with her instead of an alcoholic roommate. One of his peers says, "That's crazy. How could you miss her when you were asleep in the driveway every night?" Jeff decides to stay in treatment a few more days.

He attends AA meetings in the hospital cafeteria at night. He admits to being an alcoholic and being powerless over alcohol. He requests a female AA sponsor but is told he must have a male sponsor. His sponsor asks Jeff if he has completed step two of AA. Jeff says, "No, I am an atheist." Later, Jeff tells some peers that he is not going to change any of his friends, even though the counselor recommended that he do so. He also indicates he is not going to go to AA. The peer says, "I hear you talking the talk in group. But can you walk the walk?"

Questions

1. Why does Jeff say he only drinks socially and does not have a drinking problem? How would you respond to this and his contention that he is only in treatment to appease his wife and lawyer?

2. Jeff's wife hears the addictionologist say that Jeff has alcohol dependence. She asks you to explain alcohol dependence and alcohol abuse. How would you respond?

3. What are the stages of alcohol withdrawal? When do they typically occur? What signs and symptoms accompany each stage?

4. What is being done to prevent or minimize Jeff's withdrawal symptoms? Why is he getting thiamine?

5. Jeff's wife asks what causes Jeff to be an alcoholic. How would you respond?

6. Jeff's wife wants to know if the health care provider can give him some pills, patches, or hypnosis to help him stop smoking while he is in treatment. How would you respond?

7. Jeff says he doesn't think his pancreatitis and gastritis are related to his alcohol use. As the nurse leading the class on the

Questions (continued)

effects of alcohol on the body, what would you tell him?

8. Why did Jeff's peer say, "That's crazy. How could you miss her when you were asleep in the driveway every night?" What did his peer mean when he said, "I hear you talking the talk, but can you walk the walk?"

9. Why did Jeff need a male AA sponsor? What are the first three steps of AA's twelve-step program? How should Jeff's sponsor respond to Jeff's assertion that he is an atheist and unable to complete steps two and three? Can the treatment program require Jeff to attend AA? Can a judge

require him to attend AA as a condition of probation for his DWI charge?

10. What are the current treatments for alcohol dependence? Discuss acupuncture alpha stimulation.

11. What problem does short-term treatment pose? What treatment implications do the diagnosis of ADHD and the traits of Conduct Disorder carry?

12. What assessment information do you need to develop a nursing care plan? What nursing diagnoses and goals would you write for this client? What nursing interventions would you write?

Questions and Suggested Answers

1. Why does Jeff say he only drinks socially and does not have a drinking problem? How would you respond to this and his contention that he is only in treatment to appease his wife and lawyer? Jeff is using the most common defense mechanism: denial. It involves denying the existence of a problem and minimizing the amount of alcohol consumed. You could confront Jeff about the incongruence between what he and his wife are saying about his drinking, but he would probably just get angry with his wife. It isn't productive to confront him now. His peers will likely confront him later, which will be more effective than confrontation by the nurse. With some coaching from the nurse and/or therapist, the wife could confront Jeff later, if deemed necessary or therapeutic, in family therapy sessions.

2. Jeff's wife hears the addictionologist say that Jeff has alcohol dependence. She asks you to explain alcohol dependence and alcohol abuse. How would you respond? *Alcohol abuse* is the condition of continuing to use alcohol despite recurring social, interpersonal, and/or legal problems resulting from its use. A person with *alcohol dependence* meets the criteria for alcohol abuse, but also exhibits additional behaviors. To meet the criteria for alcohol dependence, a person must have a maladaptive pattern of alcohol use that leads to significant impairment or distress as demonstrated by three or more of the following happening at any time in the same one-year period:

1. Tolerance, which is either the need for greatly increased amounts of alcohol to achieve intoxication or greatly diminished effect with ongoing use of the same amount of alcohol

2. Withdrawal, as shown by either the usual withdrawal syndrome for alcohol or taking the same or a related substance to relieve or avoid withdrawal symptoms

3. Frequently ingesting larger amounts of alcohol over a longer period than the person intends

4. Having a persistent wish to reduce or control alcohol use or lack of success in efforts to do so

5. Spending a lot of time obtaining, using, or recovering from the effects of alcohol

6. Giving up or reducing involvement in important activities (e.g., social, work, or recreational activities) due to alcohol use

7. Continuing to use alcohol in spite of persistent or recurring physical or mental problems that seem attributable to or made worse by alcohol

Alcohol dependence can be with or without physiologic dependence, meaning with or without evidence of tolerance or withdrawal (APA, 2002).

3. What are the stages of alcohol withdrawal? When do they typically occur? What signs and symptoms accompany each stage? Blondell (2005) describes three stages of alcohol withdrawal. Stage One is minor withdrawal, which usually begins five to six hours after the client's last drink. Signs and symptoms associated with this stage include anxiety, restlessness, agitation, mild nausea, decreased appetite, sleep disturbance, facial sweating, mild tremulousness, tachycardia, and hypertension. Mild cognitive impairment might be present.

Stage Two is major withdrawal, which occurs twenty-four to seventy-two hours after the last drink. This stage is marked by restlessness, agitation, and moderate tremulousness. The client might exhibit constant eye movement, diaphoresis, nausea and vomiting, anorexia, diarrhea, tachycardia, and high systolic blood pressure (over 160 mm Hg). The client can experience alcoholic hallucinosis and disorientation, but can be reoriented. Seizure can occur; typically, it is a grand mal seizure lasting less than five minutes. Sometimes the client has two to three seizures in a row.

Stage Three, delirium tremens, can begin seventy-two to ninety-six hours after the client's last drink. The client can exhibit fever, severe hypertension, profuse sweating, marked tremulousness, and delirium. People in Stage Three can die of various causes such as head trauma, cardiovascular complications, infection, aspiration pneumonia, and fluid and electrolyte imbalances.

4. What is being done to prevent or minimize Jeff's withdrawal symptoms? Why is he getting thiamine? Jeff is receiving lorazepam and chlordiazepoxide, medications helpful in relieving or minimizing agitation and anxiety. They also prevent the client's blood pressure from becoming elevated. Blondell (2005) claims that chlordiazepoxide and diazepam (Valium), both long-acting benzodiazepams, are agents of choice in detoxifying clients, as they are effective in preventing alcohol withdrawal symptoms and delirium.

Thiamine prevents Wernicke-Korsakoff's syndrome, which occurs due to thiamine deficiency. Long-term, heavy drinkers often fail to eat a balanced diet or an adequate amount. Heavy drinkers might feel that food ruins the effects of the alcohol. Alcoholics often do not have an adequate intake of thiamine (vitamin B_1). They also fail to take vitamin supplements regularly. In addition, alcohol interferes with the active gastrointestinal (GI) transport of thiamine. In a state of chronic liver disease, there is decreased activation of thiamine pyrophosphate from thiamine and diminished capacity to store thiamine. Chronic alcoholics can become thiamine deficient; this deficiency can result in Wernicke's encephalopathy, which has a mortality rate of 10–20 percent; of those who survive, 80 percent will have Korsakoff's psychosis and require long-term institutionalization (Salen, 2001). Early symptoms of thiamine deficiency include tiredness, irritability, impaired memory, sleep disturbances, loss of appetite, abdominal pain, constipation, and chest pain; most people have no symptoms (Busschots and Vallee, 2002). Symptoms of Wernicke's encephalopathy include ocular abnormalities such as horizontal nystagmus and paralysis of the lateral rectus muscles; less frequently the pupils present as sluggish in reaction. The client could exhibit ptosis, confusion with apathy, impaired awareness of the immediate situation, spatial disorientation, inattention, and difficulty concentrating. In addition ataxia, hyperthermia from involvement of the temperature-regulating center, and hypotension could occur. Coma is sometimes the only manifestation of Wernicke's encephalopathy (Salen, 2001). Clients with chronic alcohol dependency must receive thiamine supplements; they should receive parenteral thiamine as a routine action when they present at a medical facility (Busschots and Vallee, 2002).

5. Jeff's wife asks what causes Jeff to be an alcoholic. How would you respond? The *Diagnostic and Statistical Manual of Mental Disorders* (APA, 2000) states that the risk for alcohol dependence triples or quadruples in close relatives of individuals with alcohol dependence. The greater the number of relatives with alcohol dependence, the greater the risk of a person developing the problem. In addition to genetic differences in alcoholics, environment appears to play a role; a supportive family might negate the effects of genetics. Other environmental factors include cultural attitude toward drinking and drunkenness, availability of alcohol, expectations about the effects of alcohol, personal experiences with alcohol, and stressors.

Jeff grew up in a family in which drinking was accepted and alcohol was readily available. The small-town culture split those who drank to socialize and those who went to church and did not drink and, perhaps, those who went to church and drank secretly. The culture equated being a man with being able to hold one's liquor and to keep up with fellow drinkers. You could point out to Jeff's wife that he probably has a genetic risk for alcohol dependence; moreover, the culture in which he grew up fostered the use and abuse of alcohol.

6. Jeff's wife wants to know if the health care provider can give him some pills, patches, or hypnosis to help him stop smoking while he is in treatment. How would you respond? When a client is in treatment for chemical addiction, it is a stressful time. Asking someone to stop smoking while he is trying to quit drinking is too much for one time. While others might want the client to stop smoking, it just won't happen until the client is motivated to quit himself. The groundwork for cultivating motivation is education, which the nurse can provide when the client is receptive. You also can prepare the wife for the reality that the client might never decide to give up smoking. At this point, the important issue is recovery from alcoholism and maintaining sobriety. The nurse can agree to assess the client's motivation to give up smoking and provide some education about smoking cessation.

7. Jeff says he doesn't think his pancreatitis and gastritis are related to his alcohol use. As the nurse leading the class on the effects of alcohol on the body, what would you tell him? You should advise Jeff that repetitive consumption of large amounts of alcohol has adverse effects on most of the body's organ systems. In particular, alcohol affects the GI tract, the cardiovascular system, and the nervous systems. The GI effects of alcohol abuse include gastritis, stomach or duodenal ulcers, and cirrhosis of the liver and pancreatitis (in about 15 percent of heavy drinkers). Alcohol abuse has been associated with an increased rate in some, but not all, types of cancers found in the GI tract. Some clients also develop cardiovascular problems and peripheral neuropathy alone or in combination with GI problems (APA, 2000).

8. Why did Jeff's peer say, "That's crazy. How could you miss her when you were asleep in the driveway every night?" What did his peer mean when he said, "I hear you talking the talk, but can you walk the walk?" The peer confronted Jeff about a transparent excuse for getting out of treatment. Jeff likely wants out to get a drink. Alcoholics commonly develop a sudden reason to leave treatment due to their alcohol cravings. In group therapy, peers are encouraged to confront each other when thinking errors occur.

When the peer speaks of Jeff talking the talk, but not walking the walk, he is referring to Jeff's actions. He talks as though he is in recovery, but Jeff is unwilling to do the things necessary to maintain sobriety. The peer questions Jeff's unwillingness to disassociate from his old drinking buddies and attend AA meetings.

9. Why did Jeff need a male AA sponsor? What are the first three steps of AA's twelve-step program? How should Jeff's sponsor respond to Jeff's assertion that he is an atheist and unable to complete steps two and three? Can the treatment program require Jeff to attend AA? Can a judge require him to attend AA as a condition of probation for his DWI charge? For a heterosexual male in AA, a same-gender sponsor removes the possibility of the person becoming attracted to or involved with the sponsor. A same-gender sponsor helps keep the focus on recovery.

The first step of AA's twelve-step program is, "We admitted we were powerless over alcohol and that our lives had become unmanageable." In step two, the alcoholic says, "Came to believe that a Power greater than ourselves could restore us to sanity." The sponsor will probably suggest that Jeff come up with a higher power of some sort. It does not have to be God or Buddha, but can be any sort of higher power. The third step is, "Made a decision to turn our will and our lives over to the care of God *as we understood him.*"

A treatment program in a private hospital or facility can make attendance at AA a requirement of the program. Ethically, the program must make potential clients aware of this requirement before admission. A 1999 Supreme Court decision let stand a ruling protecting the right of an atheist to refuse mandatory attendance at AA meetings as a condition for probation.

10. What are the current treatments for alcohol dependence? Discuss acupuncture and alpha stimulation. Treatment begins by getting the person to recognize that he has a problem with alcoholism, since this disease is associated with the tendency to deny the problem and its severity. Tranquilizers and sedatives are used for four to seven days to control symptoms of alcohol withdrawal. Treatment also helps people look at situations triggering abuse and assists them in developing coping skills (Reyes, 2001).

Health care providers use disulfiram (Antabuse) with some clients. When people on disulfiram drink, it causes an unpleasant reaction including throbbing head and neck pain, difficulty breathing, nausea and vomiting, sweating, flushing, tachycardia, and dizziness. This reaction can last thirty minutes to several hours. Even after stopping disulfiram, a person can experience an unpleasant reaction with alcohol ingestion for up to two weeks. Disulfiram also can cause drowsiness, depression, and erectile dysfunction (Reyes, 2001).

Health care providers also use the opiate antagonist naltrexone (ReVia) combined with a variety of psychosocial therapies. Naltrexone helps decrease the craving for alcohol. Kenna and associates (2004) posit that, although naltrexone and behavior therapy might decrease both the number of drinking days and heavy drinking as well as the time to relapse in some alcohol-dependent persons, these treatments are not effective for many other patients. Recent advances in molecular and behavior genetics are guiding the development of new drugs for the treatment of alcohol dependence.

In July 2004, the U.S. Food and Drug Administration (FDA) approved acamprosate calcium (Campral) to help maintain abstinence from alcohol in clients with alcohol dependence who were abstaining at the time the medication was initiated. Its use should comprise part of a comprehensive management program that includes psychosocial support. Acamprosate calcium, the first new drug approved for treatment of alcohol dependence in nearly ten years, is believed to restore the brain's chemical balance. Chronic alcohol intake is thought to change the normal neuronal excitation and inhibition balance; thus, acamprosate calcium interacts with neurotransmitter systems to restore normal balance. (*Pain and Central Nervous System Week,* February 7, 2005).

Acupuncture targeting the earlobes is used with alcoholics. At the very least, this treatment produces relaxation. Some nurses working in alcohol and drug treatment programs are trained to use acupuncture with alcohol-abusing and dependent clients.

Alpha stimulation involves a battery-powered unit with pads that are attached to the earlobes. The unit delivers a small current to the earlobes in order to stimulate deep relaxation. Another relaxation technique involves wearing a special helmet with flashing lights. Alcohol and other drug treatment centers also use meditation, guided imagery, and stress-reduction techniques with clients.

11. What problem does short-term treatment pose? What treatment implications do the diagnosis of ADHD and the traits of Conduct Disorder carry?

Clients in alcohol treatment programs do not possess a clear mind when coming off alcohol; many will not have a clear mind until after the initial short-term treatment program is finished. Zinn and colleagues (2004) looked at deficits in executive functioning and their impact on alcoholism treatment. They suggest developing treatment approaches that demand less of the brain's executive functions, especially in the areas of learning, reasoning, and cognitive functioning, when helping recently detoxed alcoholic clients.

In regard to modifying interventions because of behaviors associated with ADHD and traits of Conduct Disorder, the nurse needs to help Jeff learn to think before acting on an impulse. The client might need to be given directions one at a time rather than all at once. The client also might need to be taught in small increments.

At age 17, the client had problems with authority figures and rules; Jeff might still have these problems. You can assess to see if this is the case. It is important for the nurse to avoid control battles, yet hold the client to the rules. Sometimes, clients will attempt to start control battles with staff to use problems with the staff as the rationale for leaving the program.

Rose and colleagues (*Pain and Central Nervous System Week*, January 17, 2005) suggest a connection between risk for alcohol abuse and behaviors associated with Conduct Disorder. They indicate that symptoms of Conduct Disorder might suggest an opportunity to target intervention.

12. What assessment information do you need to develop a nursing care plan? What nursing diagnoses and goals would you write for this client? What nursing interventions would you write? You want to know this client's strengths and limitations so you can build on his strengths. You also want to know what successful coping mechanisms the client has used in the past, as well as any ineffective ones. You want to assess the client's physical and mental state and how ready he is to assume responsibility for attaining and maintaining a healthy state. Many clients with addiction problems are more externally controlled than internally controlled, meaning that they believe fate, luck, or some force beyond their control determines whether they will develop health problems, not their habits or behaviors. The client's mood needs to be assessed; alcohol is a depressant, and many alcoholics are depressed.

Possible nursing diagnoses are:

- Nutrition, less than required
- Ineffective coping mechanisms
- Altered role performance
- Powerlessness
- Knowledge deficit

Goals could include:

- Will maintain sobriety
- Will learn recreational skills that do not involve alcohol
- Will describe three ways to relieve stress that do not involve alcohol
- Will identify appropriate roles and behaviors as husband and father

Nursing interventions could include:

- Administer medications as ordered and assess vital signs frequently to prevent withdrawal signs and symptoms
- Encourage and provide small, frequent meals, as the alcoholic's stomach is often small from not eating

- Provide notebooks and writing instruments for journaling and twelve-step work
- Provide teaching about medication
- Provide education about harmful effects of alcohol
- Provide education about healthy ways to relieve stress
- Provide teaching about problem-solving techniques; role-model use of problem solving
- Encourage participation in AA meetings, when appropriate
- Provide and encourage recreational activities

The client's day-to-day sobriety is an important measure of his treatment success. Because the alcoholic is always recovering and never cured, evaluation must be ongoing. You must measure progress toward goals, revising them upward or downward, or changing them when appropriate, to help the client meet his goals.

References

American Psychiatric Association (APA). (2000). *Diagnostic and Statistical Manual of Mental Disorders, 4th ed.* Text Revision. Washington, DC: APA.

Blondell, R. D. (2005). "Ambulatory Detoxification of Patients with Alcohol Dependence." *American Family Physician* 71(3): 495–503.

Busschots, G. V. and P. A. Vallee. (2002). "Beriberi (Thiamine Deficiency)." http://www.emedicine.com/med/topic221.htm. Accessed March 27, 2005.

"Conduct Disorder, Alcoholism May Have Different Origins in Teens." (January 17, 2005). *Pain and Central Nervous System Week,* 12–14.

Kenna, G. A., et al. (2004). "Pharmacotherapy, Pharmacogenics, and the Future of Alcohol Dependence Treatment Part I." *American Journal of Health System Pharmacy* 61(21): 2272–2280.

"New Treatment for Alcoholism: Campral Available." (February 7, 2005). *Pain and Central Nervous System Week,* 14.

Reyes, A. (2001). "Alcohol Dependence." http://3-rx.com/alcohol-dependence/treatment.php. Accessed March 27, 2005.

Salen, P. (2001). "Wernicke Encephalopathy." http://www.emedicine.com/emerg/topic642.htm. Accessed March 27, 2005.

Zinn, S., et al. (2004). "Executive Functioning Early in Abstinence From Alcohol." *Alcohol Clinical Experimental Research* 28(9): 1338–1346.

CASE STUDY 2

Jake

GENDER

M

AGE

25

SETTING

- Inpatient residential treatment center for drug addiction

ETHNICITY

- Black American

CULTURAL CONSIDERATIONS

- Drugs
- Music
- Black American, predominantly Black American church

PREEXISTING CONDITION

COEXISTING CONDITION

COMMUNICATION

DISABILITY

SOCIOECONOMIC

- Comes from upper-middle-class family, but is homeless and penniless due to drug dependence

SPIRITUAL/RELIGIOUS

- Grew up Baptist
- Father is a minister
- Sang in choir

PHARMACOLOGIC

PSYCHOSOCIAL

LEGAL

- Using illegal substances

ETHICAL

- Should a peer report a nurse suspected of drug abuse? (both a legal and an ethical issue)

ALTERNATIVE THERAPY

- Psychodrama
- Auricular acupuncture
- Anger management

PRIORITIZATION

DELEGATION

CHEMICAL OR SUBSTANCE ABUSE

Level of difficulty: High

Overview: Requires the ability to work professionally, therapeutically, and nonjudgmentally. The nurse must be supportive of the client.

Client Profile

Jake is a 25-year-old male with a bachelor's degree in music who grew up in an upper-middle-class family. His father is the minister of a large Baptist church; his mother is a college professor. While growing up, Jake sang in the church choir and was active in the church. After college, he drifted away from the church. He took a job as a bartender and played in a band. The band members smoked marijuana and drank beer. The band manager received a gift of cocaine one Christmas and shared it with the band members. At the time, Jake was depressed because his girlfriend had left him. After "snorting" the cocaine, he felt euphoric. Soon, he and his fellow band members were using cocaine every day. The more cocaine they used, the worse the band sounded. Eventually the band split up, as no one would hire them.

One day, Jake was inventorying the bar's liquor after hours. He did a line of cocaine and then heard a knock at the door. It was the police; the officer was a former high-school classmate. After the officer left, Jake went to the bathroom; he was shocked to see white powder on his mustache. The police officer didn't arrest him or try to get him into treatment; however, Jake's father did when he discovered cash missing from the church and pawn tickets for family belongings. He thought about the changes in his son's behavior and put two and two together.

Four days into a residential drug treatment program, Jake abruptly left. He had an intense craving for cocaine. He soon found that he needed more cocaine to satisfy his cravings. Jake began calling his mother and asking for money. When she refused, he called her terrible names and blamed her for his problems. His mother's Al-Anon friends told her not to talk to him, but she was afraid to do so. Apparently, one of her Al-Anon group friends ignored her son and he committed suicide. His father told him, "Stop calling and don't come home or to the church until you've completed treatment."

Case Study

Jake admits himself to another residential drug treatment program after a new girlfriend leaves him over his cocaine use. He also has lost his bartending job. He has sold all his belongings, is overdrawn at the bank, and owes a number of people money, as well as the credit card company. He is living on the street.

The facility's screening staff call his father. Jake's father once more agrees to pay for treatment. The nurse admits Jake. Then, she asks Jake when he last did cocaine. He responds, "About eight hours ago."

There are two female clients on the unit. Jake quickly forms a friendship with one who is his age. He starts talking about moving in with her after they are discharged. She is discharged the day after Jake arrives on the unit.

The psychiatrist orders individual therapy, network therapy, education group, anger management, psychodrama, and auricular acupuncture. The psychiatrist, who also is the network therapy group leader, asks the nurse to colead the group with him. The group comprises several alcoholics, three heroin abusers, and Jake.

Jake must have a family member or friend serve as a support person in network therapy. He tells the nurse that he wants the female client who was just discharged to be his support person. He also tells the nurse that one of her colleagues—a nurse on the unit—is a drug user. He says he saw her buying cocaine in the bar in which he worked.

Questions

1. What is cocaine? Is it a stimulant or a depressant? How is it used?

2. What are the criteria for Cocaine Abuse and Cocaine Dependence? Does Jake match either of these criteria sets?

3. Would you expect this client to have unpleasant physical withdrawal symptoms? Does the withdrawal from cocaine differ from the withdrawal from heroin? If Jake begins to have symptoms of physiologic withdrawal, what question(s) would you ask him?

4. What is the major challenge the treatment team faces when a client suddenly stops using cocaine? Will Jake experience triggers to craving cocaine? What are some examples of triggers?

5. What is network therapy? How would you respond to Jake's request to have a peer who recently left treatment as his support person? Why would Jake develop a relationship with a female peer so quickly?

6. Are there any black American cultural beliefs and/or practices of which you need to be aware when working with Jake?

7. What treatment modalities are used for cocaine abuse? What medications are under study?

8. You need to teach Jake and his peers about the short-term effects of cocaine and its long-term harmful effects on the body. What are these effects?

9. What is the prevalence of cocaine use in the United States? Are there gender and race differences? What is the course of cocaine use? What causes cocaine-related deaths?

10. Jake identifies one of your coworkers as having purchased cocaine. What should you do? What are the signs of cocaine abuse?

11. You are developing a nursing care plan for this client. What nursing diagnoses and goals will you likely write? What nursing interventions would be helpful for this client?

Questions and Suggested Answers

1. What is cocaine? Is it a stimulant or a depressant? How is it used?
Cocaine is a stimulant that produces a euphoric "high" of short duration.
It comes from the leaves of the Erythroxylon coca bush. When sold on the
street, it is usually a fine, white, crystalline powder. Some street names are
coke, snow, flake, and blow, among others. It is often diluted with other
substances such as cornstarch, sugar, talcum powder, or other drugs such as
amphetamines. Pure cocaine can be lethal, as users expect it to be diluted;
unaware of the purity, they overdose and die.

The National Institute on Drug Abuse (2005) states that cocaine comes
in two chemical forms. One form is hydrochloride salt; it is a powdered
form that can be taken intranasally or dissolved in water and taken intravenously. The second form is "freebase." One form of freebase is crack
cocaine, which is "cocaine powder processed with ammonia or sodium
bicarbonate (baking soda) and water, and heated to remove the hydrochloride." The freebase forms are smoked (NIDA, 2005, 1–2). Cocaine is most
often snorted through the nose using a straw or a currency bill rolled up
like a straw, and a line of powdered cocaine. When injected intravenously,
it gives a faster high, but carries the risk of human immunodeficiency virus
(HIV) if sharing needles with HIV-infected persons. Some people mix
cocaine powder or crack with heroin to form a "speedball." Freebasing
involves smoking cocaine in a pipe; it gives an intense, but quickly disap-
pearing, high. When the high disappears, the user has an enormous craving to freebase again. Users quickly build a tolerance and have to increase
both dose and frequency (Focus Adolescent Services, 2000).

Cocaine has some legitimate medical uses. It is a schedule II drug, which
indicates its potential for abuse. Some clients enter treatment for abusing
prescription drugs containing cocaine.

**2. What are the criteria for Cocaine Abuse and Cocaine Dependence?
Does Jake match either of these criteria sets?** The *Diagnostic and Statistical
Manual of Mental Disorders* (APA, 2000) does not provide separate criteria
for abuse or dependence for the different types of substances (i.e., cocaine,
heroin, alcohol, etc.); instead, it provides general criteria. The criteria
for dependence require three or more of seven symptoms occurring at
any time during a one-year period representing a "maladaptive pattern of
substance use, leading to clinically significant impairment or distress." The
seven symptoms are

1. Tolerance
2. Withdrawal
3. Taking the substance in greater amounts over a greater period of
   time than was intended

4. Persistent desire or lack of success in cutting down or controlling use of the substance
5. Spending a lot of time in activities to get the substance
6. Giving up, or reducing time spent in, important social, work, or fun activities
7. Continuing use of the substance despite knowledge of having an ongoing or recurring physical or psychological problem, which probably was caused or made worse by the substance (APA, 2000, 197)

A diagnosis of Substance Abuse can be made if the client's symptoms have "never met the criteria for Substance Dependence for this class of substance" and the client has at least one of the four following symptoms within the same year period representing a "maladaptive pattern of substance use, leading to clinically significant impairment or distress":

1. Failing to meet major role obligations due to recurrent substance abuse
2. Repeatedly using substance in physically hazardous situations like driving an automobile under the influence of the substance
3. Recurring substance-related legal problems
4. Continuing to use in spite of ongoing or recurring social or interpersonal problems due to or exacerbated by the effects of the substance (APA, 2000, 199)

Although Jake exhibits symptoms of Substance Abuse, he would not be given this diagnosis because he meets the criteria for Substance Dependence. He likely matches criteria three through seven for Substance Dependence.

3. Would you expect this client to have unpleasant physical withdrawal symptoms? Does the withdrawal from cocaine differ from the withdrawal from heroin? If Jake begins to have symptoms of physiologic withdrawal, what question(s) would you ask him? It is possible that this client will not experience physical withdrawal symptoms. Many cocaine users, even heavy users, do not have physical withdrawal symptoms. When physical symptoms are present, they include fatigue, vivid or unpleasant dreams, sleeping a lot or a little, a greater appetite than usual, and psychomotor changes consisting of either agitated or slowed behavior. Heavy users can experience these symptoms immediately after a high or within a few hours or days of the last use.

Intense psychologic craving for cocaine is common, but the *Diagnostic and Statistical Manual of Mental Disorders* (APA, 2000) does not list it as a symptom for a diagnosis of withdrawal. It only requires that the client has stopped using cocaine, is experiencing two or more of the symptoms listed above, and some impairment or distress in some significant area of the person's life is being caused by the symptoms. Intense psychologic craving with cocaine withdrawal is a causative factor in relapse, whereas the physical symptoms in heroin withdrawal are deterrents to relapse once the client has been detoxified. The client withdrawing from heroin has physical symptoms including depressed mood, restlessness, tearing and/or nasal discharge, muscle aches, diarrhea, nausea and vomiting, dilated pupils, chills, sweating, fever, yawning, and insomnia. Withdrawal from heroin occurs approximately six to twenty-four hours after the last use.

If Jake begins to have severe physiologic withdrawal symptoms, you need to ask about other drug use. Since physiologic withdrawal symptoms from cocaine are milder and different from withdrawal from heroin and other drugs, Jake might be withdrawing from another drug in addition to cocaine. Some clients abuse both cocaine and heroin, and they often abuse alcohol as well.

4.   What is the major challenge the treatment team faces when a client suddenly stops using cocaine? Will Jake experience triggers to craving cocaine? What are some examples of triggers? The major challenge is to keep the client in treatment and prevent relapse. The client's psychologic cravings will prompt him or her to use any excuse to get out of treatment and get cocaine. Common excuses for leaving treatment include: staff members are unfair or treat the client badly; staff do not know what they are doing; or the client has urgent business and must leave the treatment center.

Some clients crave cocaine upon seeing any white powder. Jake might experience craving when pouring sugar from a cafeteria container or seeing the cook work with flour. Triggers also include being around friends they used with, being in places near or where they used, or drinking drinks they used to drink when using cocaine. If they purchased or did cocaine near a gas station or convenience store selling gasoline, the smell of gasoline might trigger an intense craving for cocaine.

5.   What is network therapy? How would you respond to Jake's request to have a peer who recently left treatment as his support person? Why would Jake develop a relationship with a female peer so quickly? Network therapy is similar to "family night" in some treatment programs but has a more specific structure. Galanter and associates (2002) characterize network therapy as having three key elements:

1. A cognitive behavioral approach
2. Involvement and support from the client's social network (e.g., spouse, family, and/or peers)
3. A community reinforcement aspect whereby clients focus on activities beyond the session context to support their rehabilitation efforts

Client can have more than one support person in therapy sessions. The person must be able to support the client after discharge in order to be a support person during network therapy. It is not appropriate to choose a one-day acquaintance or a peer undergoing treatment. You need to discuss Jake's request with the group leader. He will either tell Jake "no" or encourage him to bring it up in group therapy so his peers can confront him about the lack of wisdom of his choice. If his peers don't confront him, the group leader will have to do so in a supportive and therapeutic way. Jake's father and/or mother are his long-term supporters. If he is serious about his ex-girlfriend, he might want to ask her too. It is not unusual for people in drug rehabilitation to be impulsive and make decisions that are problematic.

Jake, a young adult, is at the Ericksonian developmental stage of intimacy versus isolation. The characteristics of this stage are "mutuality and intimacy with another person" (Frisch and Frisch, 2006, 43). One of his developmental tasks is to find a life mate. Cocaine use affects the frontal cortex of the brain; thus, it affects both judgment and the ability to think things through. As Jake is not thinking clearly at this time, it is important for you to model good decision making and teach decision-making skills.

6. Are there any black American cultural beliefs and/or practices of which you need to be aware when working with Jake? According to Antai-Otong (2002), the four major parts at the core of black American culture are "spirituality, reverence for women and older adults, family and community ties, and legacy of storytelling" (Antai-Otong, 2002, 16–17). The substance-abusing black American feeling shame and stigma can draw support from family, community, and story telling. An adult, black American male might respond well to interventions involving spirituality, reverence for women and older adults, family and community ties, and storytelling. They also would fit well with network therapy.

You need to assess Jake's status in terms of spirituality and religion as well as the other three core cultural aspects. It might seem that Jake has rejected religion and given his mother a difficult time as part of an adolescent rebellion that has continued beyond adolescence. This needs to be checked out. Anger might be behind his rejection of core cultural beliefs; it also could be related to his father being a minister. Network or individual therapy can help disclose the sources of Jake's anger, as can journaling, anger management, and psychodrama.

7. What treatment modalities are used for cocaine abuse? What medications are being studied? Cognitive Behavioral Therapy (CBT) and twelve-step work are important treatment modalities for clients with cocaine abuse. In Jake's case, CBT comprises part of network therapy. Carroll (1998) authored a manual on CBT for the National Institute on Drug Abuse, which is available online.

Narcotics Anonymous (NA) uses the twelve-step work of Alcoholics Anonymous. Drug treatment programs introduce clients to the concept of NA, often having in-house NA meetings or promoting NA meetings in the community.

Research (D'Alberto, 2004) supports the efficacy of auricular acupuncture. D'Alberto's study of eighty-two heroin and cocaine addicts found that, at the end of eight weeks of treatment, more subjects who underwent acupuncture were testing free of drugs. In addition, drug treatment centers have been using acupuncture since the 1970s to alleviate withdrawal symptoms and cravings, with self-reports of success (Focus Adolescent Services, 2000). Some acupuncture treatments use five specific points on the outer ear. Performing acupuncture requires specialized training; in some treatment facilities, nurses are trained in auricular acupuncture.

Psychodrama is a technique that allows clients to try out new, and hopefully more effective, behaviors and roles in a supportive environment (ASGPP, 2006). It requires a director who has been trained in psychodrama techniques (i.e., a leader), auxiliary egos (i.e., people who play the roles of significant others), a protagonist (i.e., the person working out an issue), and an audience of peers. The director guides the group through a warm up and then an action sequence using a variety of techniques. One technique involves reversing roles back and forth to gain insight.

Carroll and associates (2004) studied the use of disulfiram (Antabuse) to treat clients abusing cocaine. Disulfiram, which has been used in the treatment of alcohol abuse for some time, is believed to alter clients' subjective and physiologic response to cocaine. According to Miller (2005), this study found that subjects taking disulfiram were less likely to relapse than those getting placebo, while those undergoing cognitive behavior therapy were less likely to relapse than those getting interpersonal psychotherapy.

Another drug, an anti-seizure drug called GVG (gamma vinyl-GABA), is being tested on animals in the United States for possible use in the treatment of cocaine addiction. GVG is approved for seizure prevention in Europe, but is not yet marketed in the United States.

An article in *Nursing* (2004) reports that researchers are investigating a number of drugs approved for other purposes for potential applications in treating clients recovering from cocaine addiction. Some of the twenty-one different drugs being studied are fluoxetine (Prozac), venlafaxine (Effexor), baclofen, tiagabine, topiramate, methylphenidate (Ritalin), amantadine, ondansetron, and propranolol. This article (*Nursing*, 2004, 31) states, "Researchers believe that within 5 years, one of the drugs currently under study will become the first to win FDA [Food and Drug Administration] approval for cocaine dependency."

8. You need to teach Jake and his peers about the short-term effects of cocaine and its long-term harmful effects on the body. What are these effects? When cocaine is taken in small amounts, there is a short-lasting feeling of euphoria. The client also feels energetic, talkative, and alert, with heightened sensations of sound, sight, and touch. The client also might experience a decreased need for food and sleep as well as restlessness, irritability, anxiety, and paranoia. Some users exhibit depression when not under the influence of the drug (Focus Adolescent Services, 2000).

Cocaine use damages the brain, particularly the prefrontal cortex. It affects decision-making abilities and judgment, as it comprises the executive decision thinking part of the brain. Phoenix House Foundation Research Director James. J. Dahl ("Collaboration between Phoenix House," 2005, 4) says this finding "is consistent with the therapeutic community model of not giving people decision-making duties during the first three-to-six months of treatment."

The blood-pressure elevations in cocaine use can weaken or rupture cerebral blood vessels, causing stroke, coma, or death. Cocaine can cause cardiac arrhythmias and heart attack.

Damage to the body can be related to how the cocaine is ingested. Smoke from crack cocaine or freebasing can cause irritation to lung tissue, coughing, and chronic respiratory tract pain as well as respiratory failure. Snorting cocaine can cause damage to vessels in the nose and nasal tissue.

9. What is the prevalence of cocaine use in the United States? Are there gender and race differences? What is the course of cocaine use? What causes cocaine-related deaths? According to 2002 data (NIDA, 2005), there are 1.5 million people in the United States who could be identified as cocaine abusers or dependent on cocaine and 2 million who could be classified as cocaine users. The highest rate of cocaine use occurs in adults age 18 to 25, with males more likely to use than females. NIDA (2005, 1) also reports that the estimated rate of cocaine use was highest for American Indians or Alaskan Natives (2.0 percent), followed by black Americans (1.6 percent), white Americans (0.8 percent), Hispanics (0.8 percent), Native Hawaiians and Pacific Islanders (0.6 percent), and Asians (0.2 percent).

The half-life of cocaine is about thirty to fifty minutes; thus, frequent dosing is required to maintain a feeling of euphoria (i.e., "a high"). There are several patterns of use, including chronic daily use and binge use. Binge use can be heavy use over the weekend or one or two weekdays separated by days of nonuse. Chronic daily use can involve use throughout the day or for only a few hours a day. Intravenous use of cocaine and smoking of cocaine seem to be associated with progression from use to abuse or dependence in weeks to months. Intranasal use can lead to abuse or dependence, but it usually occurs over months to years. Tolerance does occur, so users need to increase doses to get the desired effect. Tolerance brings a decrease in pleasurable effects and an increase in dysphoric effects.

Focus Adolescent Services (2000) indicates that cocaine use can result in emergency situations such as hypertensive crisis, acute myocardial infarction and ventricular arrhythmias necessitating immediate treatment. Further, drug-related deaths are most likely to be from cocaine, according to medical examiners reports. Hospital emergency and drug treatment centers generally find cocaine abusers to be the group most seeking emergency care.

Cocaine also causes hyperthermia, which can result in death, according to researchers (Crandall et al., 2002, 784). They found that cocaine "elevates body temperature by impairing the body's ability to increase skin-blood flow, to sweat and to perceive excessive heat stress." According to these researchers, more studies could shed light on the exact mechanisms involved, making it possible to identify new drugs that can reduce cocaine-induced hyperthermia.

Overdose can cause death when a user unknowingly ingests pure cocaine, looses track of dosage, or is allergic to cocaine or additives to the cocaine.

10. Jake identifies one of your coworkers as having purchased cocaine. What should you do? What are the signs of cocaine abuse? This is a real-life scenario. It happens, and it could happen to you. You should talk to your supervisor. If enough clues indicate that this nurse is on drugs, an intervention might be planned in which the suspected nurse sits and listens to people who care about him talk about their feelings and what they have observed. The nurse will be asked to go into treatment at another facility. In most states, the nurse can agree to enter a peer assistance program that administers random drug screens and provides a nurse advocate. If the nurse refuses, he must be reported to the state Board of Nursing, which will investigate the matter. If a charge of drug usage is substantiated, action can be taken against the nursing license. You should be familiar with your state's peer assistance program for nurses.

You should observe the peer for signs of cocaine abuse and be alert to these signs in other coworkers. The signs of cocaine use are

- Change in school grades or behavior or work performance
- Red or bloodshot eyes
- Nasal discharge or sniffing
- Change in eating or sleeping patterns
- Change in friends
- Withdrawn, depressed, tired
- Decreased attention to personal appearance
- Loss of interest in school, family, or activities
- Asking for money or borrowing or pawning

11. You are developing a nursing care plan for this client. What nursing diagnoses and goals will you likely write? What nursing interventions would be helpful for this client? Potential nursing diagnoses include:

- At risk for injury related to cocaine use
- Knowledge deficit related to harmful effects of cocaine use

- Interrupted family processes or readiness for enhanced family processes, depending on assessment of family dynamics
- Noncompliance with treatment regimen related to psychological drug craving

Goals include:

- No evidence of cocaine use or use of other addictive substances
- Negative random urine screens
- 100 percent compliance with treatment regimen
- 100 percent attendance at all scheduled group and individual therapy sessions
- Will verbalize a commitment to work in recovery and remain in recovery one day at a time
- Will express a feeling of being comfortable with family relationships or that they are improving
- Will describe a plan for avoiding drug contacts and triggers for drug use
- Will demonstrate progress in twelve-step work
- Will attend NA meetings as outlined in treatment plan

Nursing interventions could include the following:

- Build a trusting therapeutic relationship by being honest, not promising anything that is impossible to deliver, and using therapeutic communication techniques and compassion
- Set clear limits with client, ensuring client knows the facility/unit rules and policies, and hold client to these rules and policies
- Provide positive reinforcement for following rules, policies, and treatment regimen
- Be consistent with the team members in interpreting the treatment program, rules, and policies; client will not benefit from special favors or being able to manipulate staff
- Treat client with respect by using client's preferred name and letting client know that the respect remains even if when he is not doing what is appropriate
- Provide scheduled and as-needed medication in a timely fashion
- Listen to client, and use techniques such as reflection and summarizing to let him know you hear what he is saying
- Provide self-esteem-building opportunities, showing client he has value and worth; help client increase self-esteem internally from positive self-verbalizations rather than externally
- Assist client in finding appropriate leisure activities and developing talents
- Help client feel some control by giving him responsibility on the unit when he is ready (e.g., lead the community group discussion

[under supervision] or take a vote among peers as to which movie to see)
- Observe client for any opportunities to obtain drugs and monitor for signs and symptoms of drug usage while in hospital
- Assist client in building a plan to prevent relapse

References

American Psychiatric Association (APA). (2000). *Diagnostic and Statistical Manual of Mental Disorders, 4th ed.* Text Revision. Washington, DC: APA.

American Society of Group Psychotherapy and Psychodrama (ASGPP). (2006). "General Information about Psychodrama." http://www.asgpp.org/pdrama1.htm. Accessed January 21, 2006.

Antai-Otong, D. (2002). "Culturally Sensitive Treatment of African Americans with Substance-Related Disorders." *Journal of Psychosocial Nursing and Mental Health Services* 40(7): 14–21.

Carroll, K. M. (1998). *A Cognitive-Behavioral Approach: Treating Cocaine Addiction.* National Institute on Drug Abuse NIH Publication No. 98-4308. Available at http://www.drugabuse.gov/TXManuals/CBT/CBT1.html.

Carroll, K. M., et al. (2004). "Efficacy of Disulfiram and Cognitive Behavior Therapy in Cocaine-Dependent Outpatients: A Randomized Placebo-Controlled Trial." *Archives of General Psychiatry* 61(3): 264–272.

Collaboration between Phoenix House, NYU Yields Critical Data on Cocaine Addiction. (2005). *Alcoholism and Drug Abuse Weekly* 17(10): 1–8.

Crandall, C. G., et al. (June 4, 2002). "Cocaine Abuse in Warm Environments Impairs Body's Perception of Heat, Ability to Sweat—And Can Be Lethal." *Annals of Internal Medicine* 136(11): 785–791.

D'Alberto, A. (2004). "Auricular Acupuncture in the Treatment of Cocaine/Crack Abuse: A Review of the Efficacy, the Use of the National Acupuncture Detoxification Association Protocol, and the Selection of Sham Points." *Journal of Alternative and Complementary Medicine* 16(6): 985–1000.

Focus Adolescent Services. (2000). "Cocaine Abuse and Addiction." http://www.focusas.com/Cocaine.html. Accessed January 21, 2006.

Frisch, N. C. and Frisch, L. E. (2006). *Psychiatric Mental Health Nursing, 3d ed.* Albany, NY: Thomson Delmar Learning.

Galanter, M., et al. (2002). "Network Therapy for Cocaine Abuse: Use of Family and Peer Supports." *American Journal on Addictions* 11(2): 161–166.

"Kicking the Habit with Familiar Drugs." (2004). *Nursing* 34(11): 31.

Miller, K. E. (2005). "Disulfiram, Behavior Therapy in Cocaine Dependency." *American Family Physician* 71(1): 163.

National Institute on Drug Abuse (NIDA). (2005). *Research Report Series—Cocaine Abuse and Addiction.* http://www.drugabuse.gov/ResearchReports/Cocaine/cocaine2.html. Accessed June 5, 2006.

CASE STUDY 3

Caroline

GENDER

F

AGE

20

SETTING

- Inpatient residential treatment center

ETHNICITY

- White American

CULTURAL CONSIDERATIONS

PREEXISTING CONDITION

- Anorexia

COEXISTING CONDITION

- Anorexia

COMMUNICATION

DISABILITY

SOCIOECONOMIC

- Upper class

PHARMACOLOGIC

PSYCHOSOCIAL

LEGAL

- Illegal drug use
- Liability for client's safety

ETHICAL

ALTERNATIVE THERAPY

PRIORITIZATION

DELEGATION

CHEMICAL OR SUBSTANCE ABUSE (HEROIN)

Level of difficulty: High

Overview: Requires assessment of the health and well-being of a young girl who has been court-ordered to receive treatment for heroin abuse, has run away, and has been returned to the facility. The client has a past history of residential treatment for Anorexia Nervosa.

Client Profile

Caroline is a 20-year-old college student from an affluent family who lives in the suburbs. Her parents are community leaders. Her younger sister is the "good one" in the family, while Caroline fluctuates between the roles of "princess" and "black sheep" of the family. Caroline's parents love her and try to give her everything she wants. In addition to an allowance of $300 a week, Caroline has a trust fund. She frequently tests her parents' patience by staying out later than allowed and not calling, threatening to run away if she can't do what she wants, skipping school, and getting bad grades even though she is smart.

Her parents once put her into residential treatment for threatening to run away from home and her anorexic behavior. Her eating improved, as did her behavior, and her parents got her admitted to college. There, she joined a society and partied more than studied, but she managed to stay in school. Recently, she was picked up for underage drinking; the police also discovered heroin and drug paraphernalia in her possession. This is her first drug charge, although she has been using heroin for about a year. During that time, she spent all her money, manipulated her parents for more money, and even secretly stole cash from them. The parents, who now have to go to court with her, had no idea she was using the money for drugs, thinking instead she was buying designer clothes and accessories.

The judge mandates Caroline to residential treatment for drug abuse and probation for one year. She must participate in individual and family therapy during that year, do 1,000 hours of community service, and pay court costs and a fine.

Case Study

Caroline runs away from the residential drug treatment center after one week and goes home. She tells her parents, "The treatment is stupid, none of the staff know what they are doing, the food is awful and makes me sick, and the bed is worn out." Her father brings her back to the center and tells her she must stay and complete her treatment. She begs him to find her a different treatment program or let her come home for a while before going into treatment, but her father holds firm.

The admitting nurse begins the readmission process. The nurse weighs Caroline and finds she weighs 102 pounds and is 5 feet 8 inches tall. Caroline says to the admitting nurse, "You know this program sucks, and I bet you can tell my Dad about a better program that I could go to." The nurse does not answer and continues checking her vital signs. Caroline says, "Well you don't have to test my urine, I wasn't out long enough to do any drugs." Caroline's father says, "I believe she came straight home, and she has not been out of my sight since then." The unit policy is to search all clients who enter the program, do a body check, remove all contraband, confiscate items the client could use to inflict self-harm, and do a urine drug screen.

Physician's orders are to readmit the client to the program and the nurse serves as a coleader in a drug education group where the health care provider, who is an addictionologist, serves as the leader and sometimes leads the community group as well.

In one group session, Caroline hangs her leather coat carefully over a chair so the designer label shows for the rest of the group to see. After group, Caroline calls her boyfriend, who used heroin with her during the past year, and asks him to come visit her. She tells the group, she is going to try to get him into treatment. The nurse confronts Caroline on the coat issue and about her idea to get the boyfriend into treatment.

Questions

1. Why did the admitting nurse ignore Caroline's statements criticizing the treatment program? If you were the admitting nurse, would you ignore this statement? Is there a better way to respond?

2. Should you have Caroline's urine tested for drugs? Why or why not?

3. What are the likely reasons Caroline ran away from the residential treatment program?

4. If this client experiences withdrawal from heroin, when might you expect this to occur? What criteria would the client have to meet for the health care provider to diagnose the client with Opioid Withdrawal?

5. The client's parents ask you, "What is heroin? What is opium? What is an opioid? How does heroin relate to opium?" What would you tell them? How is heroin used?

6. What are people with heroin (opioid) dependence like in terms of ethnicity, culture, age, and gender?

7. Why do you think heroin use is shifting from the inner city to suburbia? Why are girls like Caroline increasingly becoming users?

8. Clients come from diverse ethnic and sociocultural backgrounds (e.g., affluent,

young, white American female versus poor, middle-aged, black American male). How might your care vary for one group versus another?

9. What information should your teaching on heroin cover?

10. What are the current treatments for Heroin Addiction and Dependence?

11. In one group session, Caroline hangs her leather coat carefully over a chair so the designer label shows for everyone in the group to see. What would you say to her, if anything, about this?

12. Caroline tells the group that she is going to try to get her boyfriend, who used heroin with her over the past year, into treatment at the same facility. What would you do or say to this client about her idea?

13. What ethical and/or legal issues must you keep in mind when working with this client?

14. What assessments do you need to do to develop a nursing care plan for this client? What nursing diagnoses will you likely write for this client? What goals do you think you might write for this client?

15. What nursing interventions would be most helpful for this client?

Questions and Suggested Answers

1.   Why did the admitting nurse ignore Caroline's statements? If you were the admitting nurse, would you ignore this statement? Is there a better way to respond? The nurse does not want to discuss other, and possibly better, programs because the client needs to be in treatment now. If the nurse defends the program, a control battle and argument could occur about the program's good and bad aspects. Admission is not the time to do a program critique or evaluation.

Some nurses might say in a kind, matter-of-fact voice, "Caroline, this is where you need to be right now. You will have the chance to bring up things you think need changing in community meeting, and you can evaluate the program when you leave. Many good changes come from clients' comments and concerns. Let's focus now on getting you admitted." This statement lets the client know that the nurse supports the admission, values the client's input at the appropriate time, indicates there will be opportunities for input, and solicits her help in the admission process.

Remember, the tone of voice, the facial expression, and the body posture of the nurse are just as important (or more important) than the words used. Some nurses use just one tone of voice. It is good to practice varying your voice tone so you can select the most therapeutic one. At times, softness of voice is required; at other times, a no-nonsense tone is therapeutic.

2.   Should you have Caroline's urine tested for drugs? Why or why not? You must have Caroline's urine checked for drugs. Treatment facility policy requires testing of all clients on admission and whenever clients leave and then return to the facility. Caroline must be held to the policies of the facility and the rules of the unit or program. All clients, including this one, need limits to stay safe and feel secure. Also, you have a legal and ethical obligation to follow the treatment facility policies. In case of a lawsuit or client death, you will have a difficult time defending your actions in court if you do not consistently comply with polices and rules. In fact, you could be held partially or totally liable for whatever happened to the client.

3.   What are the likely reasons Caroline ran away from the residential treatment program? Children and adolescents admitted to a treatment facility will test the limits and resist the rules and structure of the unit. They commonly tell their parents or guardians that the program is awful in order to go home. They will complain about staff stupidity, terrible food, and awful beds. Adolescents use similar tactics to justify skipping school or not doing homework. The drug-abusing client might try to get out of the program for the most powerful reason of all: to use drugs. Drug cravings will prompt them to try anything.

4. If this client experiences withdrawal from heroin, when might you expect this to occur? What criteria would the client have to meet for the health care provider to diagnose the client with Opioid Withdrawal? Withdrawal from heroin or any of the opioids occurs after the client has had long-term, heavy opioid use or after the client is given an opioid antagonist such as naloxone (Narcan) or naltrexone (ReVia) after a long period of use. To meet the diagnosis of Opioid Withdrawal, the client must have either stopped or reduced significant opioid use that lasted several weeks or more. There are a number of possible signs and symptoms of withdrawal syndrome. The client must exhibit at least three of nine symptoms, occurring within minutes to several days after stopping or reducing the drug or getting an opioid antagonist. These signs and symptoms must cause significant distress or impairment in an important area of functioning, and they must not be due to another medical condition or mental disorder. According to the *Diagnostic and Statistical Manual of Mental Disorders* (APA, 2000), signs and symptoms include:

- Dysphoric mood
- Inability to sleep
- Complaint of muscles aching
- Tearing or nasal discharge
- Gooseflesh, dilated pupils, or sweating
- Diarrhea
- Frequent yawning
- Elevated body temperature
- Nausea and/or vomiting

Clients will begin heroin withdrawal symptoms within six to twelve hours after their last dose because it is a short-acting drug. Symptoms will peak in one to three days and subside over five to seven days. Those who have experienced acute withdrawal from Heroin describe it as extremely uncomfortable and often resume its use and schedule use to avoid withdrawal.

Chronic symptoms include insomnia, dysphoria, anhedonia, and drug craving. It is important to get as accurate a picture as possible of the client's last use of the drug as well as his or her history of drug use. Clients tend to understate drug use, lie about it, or deny it. Thus, the nurse must be alert for possible heroin withdrawal.

5. The client's parents ask you, "What is heroin? What is opium? What is an opioid? How does heroin relate to opium?" What would you tell them? How is heroin used? Opium is extracted from the poppy plant, then it is refined to make morphine. Next, it is refined again to make heroin. In a pure form, heroin is a fine, white, granular powder; however, color can vary depending on the additives used to dilute it and how pure or how processed it is.

Heroin can be rose, grey, brown, or black in color. Although pure heroin has become more available and popular, the usual street drug is cut with substances such as powdered milk, starch, sugar, or quinine (NIDA, 2005). Users, both novice and veteran, can experience problems by not knowing the purity of the drug. When they get a purer form than they have been using but ingest the same amount, they can overdose accidentally.

Heroin is illegal and highly addictive. It also is the most rapidly acting of the opiates (NIDA, 2005).

Heroin can be smoked, snuffed, or injected. Injecting heroin is the most dangerous route because the drug reaches the brain quickly and in larger amounts than when taken in other ways. People using heroin for the first time describe feeling extroverted and being able to talk easily to others, even if they normally can't. Sexual performance might be heightened. Gordon (2002) found that 39 percent of users in one treatment facility had used heroin by injecting it; 18 percent had mixed intravenous use and snorting.

6. What are people with heroin (opioid) dependence like in terms of ethnicity, culture, age, and gender? Currently, the male-to-female ratio of heroin abusers is about three to one in the United States. According to Stoil (1999), from 1993 to 1999 more than 33 percent of admissions for heroin treatment involved individuals age 40 and older; the average client was 35 years old. Most were male and either black American or Hispanic.

According to Rosenker (2002), the demographics are changing. He found that young heroin addicts admitted to an adolescent treatment center in 1995 were almost all male; by 2002, twice as many females were being admitted for treatment of Heroin Addiction. He characterizes the new generation of heroin users as affluent, young, and from suburbia.

7. Why do you think heroin use is shifting from the inner city to suburbia? Why are girls like Caroline increasingly becoming users? Rosenker (2002) and Gordon (2002) agree on the profile of today's heroin users. At the same time teens of wealthy parents have moved to suburban areas of the country, the price of heroin has fallen and its purity has risen. Rosenker (2002, 1) describes them as "overly independent and having limitless life-styles." They have fewer parental limits and sufficient freedom and money to engage in drug use without being detected.

The rise in heroin use among adolescent and young adult women might be attributable to the weight loss said to occur with heroin use. They gain the gaunt model look that fits with society's of beauty. Some individuals who suffer from Anorexia Nervosa or Bulimia can achieve the ideal weight loss they seek without drawing attention to themselves with the usual behaviors associated with those disorders.

Perhaps yet another reason for young people doing heroin is the tremendous interest and investment of money by this group in music, concerts, and entertainment, especially that of rock bands and pop icons, which are known to promote the appeal of Heroin (Rosenker, 2002).

8. Clients come from diverse ethnic and sociocultural backgrounds (e.g., affluent, young, white American female versus poor, middle-aged, black American male). How might your care vary for one group versus another? Antai-Otong (2002, 16) states, "Ethnicity refers to a sense of identity or connectedness within a community or social group that shares values, beliefs, goals, and mores." Culture carries a set of influences shaping members' health practices and responses, including mental functioning, perception of health and illness, and development of symptoms. For example, Antai-Otong (2002) identifies the four major parts of the core of black American culture as spirituality, reverence for women and older adults, family and community ties, and the legacy of storytelling. The substance-abusing black American feeling shame and stigma can draw support from family, community, and storytelling. Thus, a middle-aged black American male might respond well to interventions involving spirituality, reverence for women and older adults, family and community ties, and storytelling whereas a white American female adult might not. She likely draws from other sources of strength and support.

It is helpful to assess the role of spirituality and religion in the client's life. Then, interventions can be individualized based on these findings. Diversity of cultures, beliefs, and practices in a treatment group can be therapeutic, helping members work through issues with new input and support. It also can cause confrontation regarding maladaptive practices and beliefs. Nurses can work with clients from other ethnic and cultural groups, if the client's best interests remain uppermost and the focus is on being therapeutic.

9. What information should your teaching on heroin cover? A 1998 survey on drug use found that 2.4 million people had used heroin at some time during their life (NIDA, 2005). In addition, almost 130,000 respondents reported using heroin within the month before the survey; approximately 81,000 people began using in 1997. Between 1991 and 1996, admissions to emergency departments involving recent heroin use more than doubled, with a fourfold increase in persons age 12 to17.

Heroin is one of the most addictive drugs. Even after just one use, the pull of addiction can be felt. Many feel a person can be addicted from the first use. Some people feel you only get addicted if you inject heroin; however, snorting or smoking lead to addiction, too.

Heroin's effects last about six hours; then, addicts begin to feel bad. One day later, their bones hurt and they feel sick; by day two or three, they will do anything to get more heroin.

Heroin users build a tolerance to the drug. They spend much of their time finding money and buying the drug. Heroin-dependent people may sell or hock all their belongings and even those of family and friends to buy heroin, spiraling downward financially until they have nothing and are on the street. Heroin-dependent people will trade sex for heroin when they run out of other resources or they are under the influence.

Use of heroin over a long period of time not only builds up a high tolerance to the drug, but also makes withdrawal likely when it is abruptly discontinued. Once dependence occurs, it typically continues for many years with only brief periods of abstinence. Eventually, 20–30 percent will achieve long-term abstinence.

The mortality rate among heroin addicts is thirty times greater than that occurring in the general population (Church of Scientology, 2004). Causes of death are as follows: 5 percent suicide, 15 percent overdose, 15 percent accidents, 30 percent murder, and 35 percent illness. Many overdoses are not reported, as most do not seek medical attention. Sporer cited in Burris, Norland and Edlin (1999, 238) states, "Acute heroin overdose is a common daily experience . . . and accounts for many preventable deaths." He advises that most overdoses occur at home in the company of others; most commonly, the overdose involves the use of alcohol and other drugs. Heroin users who overdose are, on average, in their late 20s to 30s, have used heroin five to ten years, and have a significant dependence. Since death from an overdose occurs one to three hours after drug use, more deaths could be prevented with timely emergency care.

10. What are the current treatments for Heroin Addiction and Dependence?
Over the past thirty years, methadone has been used to treat Heroin Addiction and Dependence. Methadone, which is taken by mouth, suppresses narcotic withdrawal symptoms for twenty-four to thirty-six hours. Methadone lasts four to six times longer than heroin, so it can be taken once a day. Further, methadone can relieve heroin cravings, a major reason for relapse (NIDA, 2005). Long-acting methadone (LAMM), which has an effect for up to seventy-two hours, also is taken orally.

One of the newer, less common treatments for Heroin Dependence is the naltrexone implant. Hulse and associates (2004) described a study they did in which they collected blood level data from two groups of subjects. One group of ten subjects (seven females and three males) received a 1.7 g-naltrexone implant; a second subject group of twenty-four people (eleven females and thirteen males) got 3.4 g. Subjects with the 1.7 implant had naltrexone levels high enough to extend coverage out for 90–160 days and those getting 3.4 kept levels high enough to extend coverage out 188–297 days depending on the blood naltrexone levels desired (1 ng/ml or 2 ng/ml).

Buprenorphine has been proposed as a treatment for Heroin Dependence. Research is being conducted to justify effectiveness. Cognitive, family, and individual therapy are most often used in combination with methadone, naltrexone, or buprenorphine.

11. In one group session, Caroline hangs her leather coat carefully over a chair so the designer label shows for everyone in the group to see. What would you say to her, if anything, about this? Caroline wants to tell everyone she can afford an expensive jacket. Perhaps her self-esteem and self-concept are low; this is one way in which she can prove her worth. While this is a common behavior among adolescents and young adults, it is impossible to know definitively why Caroline turned the label so others could read it. However, it is never safe to jump to conclusions about someone else's behavior. One of her peers might confront her, or the group might share their feelings about Caroline and her designer clothes.

If the problem is self-esteem or ego need, you want to be therapeutic and not lower her self-esteem any more. Perhaps you could talk with her individually and say something like, "Caroline, I noticed that you turned your jacket label so we could all see it. What is that about?" If she gets angry, you might say, "Just think about it."

12. Caroline tells the group that she is going to try to get her boyfriend, who used heroin with her over the past year, into treatment at the same facility. What would you do or say to this client about her idea? There might be a rule against clients having significant others in the treatment program at the same time. If such a rule exists, you could let her know about it and suggest that she help herself first. If no rule exists, it is preferable for peers to give the client feedback or confront her. This client is at Erickson's stage of intimacy versus isolation. The influence and opinions of peers are more important to her than those of authority figures. As the nurse coleader of the group, you might say, "Does anyone have any feedback for Caroline about her idea of getting her boyfriend into therapy with her?" You might even encourage each person in group to give her feedback. Knowledgeable peers will recognize that Caroline is focusing on her boyfriend and taking care of him rather than focusing on her own recovery. If no one mentions the detrimental effect on her own recovery, you might say, "Sometimes people take the emphasis off their own therapy and focus on someone else's. When they do, they aren't taking care of their own needs. Can anyone give an example of this?" These prompts might get Caroline's peers to confront her, or at least share their insights on her behavior.

13. What ethical and/or legal issues must you keep in mind when working with this client? Confidentiality is always an issue. It is unethical and illegal for the nurse or other health care workers to breach confidentially. The nurse and other staff must be alert to the possibility that the client is using while undergoing treatment. An article in *Managed Care Weekly Digest* (2004) describes the overdose death of a client at a treatment center. There were clues that the client had been taking drugs while in treatment. This and other clues were evident and the court said the drug treatment center could have done more to prevent the client's death.

14. What assessments do you need to do to develop a nursing care plan for this client? What nursing diagnoses will you likely write for this client? What goals do you think you might write for this client? You will need to do a physical and mental assessment. The client might have some physical signs and symptoms related to Opium Withdrawal, Anorexia Nervosa, or other causes; you do not want to miss them by focusing only on psychosocial assessments. You also need to ascertain when the client last had heroin, what her pattern of drug use was, and if she is a polydrug user. You should do a review of body systems. The client also needs to be assessed for self-esteem; body image; self-concept; orientation; judgment and insight; motivation for treatment compliance; perception of family dynamics; current significant relationships and whether or not the client has been, or is currently, sexually active; leisure and other interests; and strengths and limitations.

Possible nursing diagnoses include:

- Risk for self-harm
- Knowledge deficit
- Nutrition less than body requirements
- Body image disturbed
- Self-esteem chronically low

Goals would include:

- No evidence of use of heroin or other addictive substances
- No loss of weight, with a weight gain to within normal range for height
- 100 percent compliance with treatment regimen
- 100 percent attendance at all scheduled group and individual therapy sessions as scheduled
- Will verbalize a commitment to work in recovery and remain in recovery one day at a time
- Will feel comfortable with family relationships or feel they are improving
- Will describe a plan for avoiding drug contacts and triggers for drug use

15. What nursing interventions would be most helpful for this client? The following nursing interventions would be helpful:

- Build a trusting, therapeutic relationship by being honest, not promising anything you cannot deliver, using therapeutic communication techniques, and showing compassion
- Set clear limits; make certain client is aware of the facility rules and policies, and hold the client to them
- Provide positive reinforcement for following rules, policies, and treatment regimen

- Be consistent with team members in interpreting the treatment program and its rules and policies; avoid special favors or being manipulated
- Treat the client with respect by using her preferred name; let her know that you respect her even when she is not doing what is appropriate
- Provide scheduled and as-needed medication in a timely fashion
- Listen to client, and use techniques such as reflection and summarizing to let her know that you hear what she is saying
- Weigh client at regular intervals, and pay attention to food and fluid intake as well as exercise, laxatives use, or anorexic behaviors
- Provide assertiveness training via an assertiveness group and/or individual work
- Provide self-esteem-building opportunities, help client know that she is valuable and has worth, and work with her to get more self-esteem internally from positive self-verbalizations rather than externally
- Assist client in finding appropriate leisure activities and developing talents
- Help client feel some control by giving her more responsibility when she can handle it (e.g., lead community group discussion [under supervision] or take a vote among peers as to which movie to see)
- Observe client for any opportunities to obtain drugs, and monitor for signs and symptoms of drug use while in treatment
- Assist client in building a plan to prevent relapse

References

American Psychiatric Association (APA). (2000). *Diagnostic and Statistical Manual of Mental Disorders, 4th ed.* Text Revision. Washington, DC: APA.

Antai-Otong, D. (2002). "Culturally Sensitive Treatment of African Americans with Substance Related Disorders." *Journal of Psychosocial Nursing* 40(7): 14–20.

Burris, S. J., J. Norland, and B. R. Edlin. (2001). "Legal Aspects of Providing Naloxone to Heroin Users in the United States." *International Journal of Drug Policy* 12: 237–248.

Church of Scientology. (2004). "Heroin: Death in the Blood." http://www.drugs-information.org. Accessed May 1, 2005.

Gordon, S. M. (2002). "Surprising Data on Young Heroin Users." *The Brown Child and Adolescent University Behavioral Letter* 18(11): 1–3.

Hulse, G. K., et al. (2004). "Blood Naltrexone and 6β-Naltrexol Levels Following Naltrexone Implant: Comparing Two Naltexone Implants." *Addiction Biology* 9(1): 69–76.

Kohn, C. and C. W. Henderson. (July 12, 2004). "Ruling Says Drug Treatment Center Could Have Done More to Prevent Death. *Managed Care Weekly Digest*, 74–76.

National Institute on Drug Abuse (NIDA). (2005). "Heroin Abuse and Addiction." NIH Publication No. 05-4165. Available online at www.nida.nih.gov/Research.Reports/heroin/Heroin.html.

Rosenker, D. C. (2002). "Special Report: Worrying New Trends in Heroin Use: Heroin Reaches the Well to Do Population." *The Brown Child and Adolescent University Behavioral Letter* 18(11): 1–3.

Stoil, M. J. (1999). "Treatment Policy—What Treatment Policy?" *Behavioral Health Management* 19(5): 6–8.

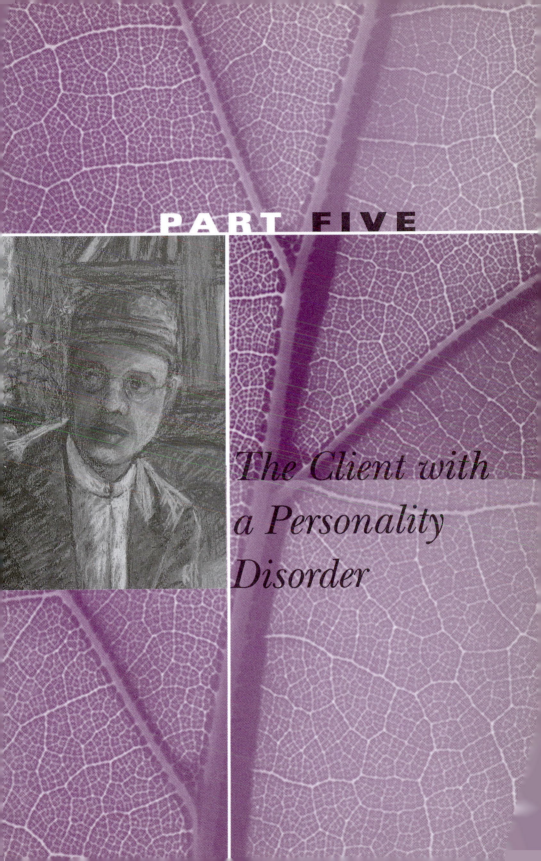

PART FIVE

The Client with a Personality Disorder

CASE STUDY 1

Martha

GENDER

F

AGE

28

SETTING

- Medical unit of a medical surgical hospital

ETHNICITY

- White American

CULTURAL CONSIDERATIONS

PREEXISTING CONDITION

COEXISTING CONDITION

COMMUNICATION

DISABILITY

SOCIOECONOMIC

SPIRITUAL/RELIGIOUS

PHARMACOLOGIC

PSYCHOSOCIAL

- "Splitting" contributes to impaired social interaction

LEGAL

ETHICAL

ALTERNATIVE THERAPY

PRIORITIZATION

- Preventing client from self-harm

DELEGATION

DIFFICULT

PERSONALITY DISORDERS

Level of difficulty: High

Overview: Requires an understanding of the concept of "splitting," critical thinking, skill in dealing with intense emotional responses, collaboration, and strict compliance with rules and limits. The nurse must plan in-service training on the care of clients with Borderline Personality Disorder, identifying both a presenter and critical content.

Client Profile

Martha is a 28-year-old white American female with a long history of Borderline Personality Disorder (BPD). She has been in individual therapy with several psychotherapists, but none for long. She has a history of suicidal attempts and self-mutilation. She has cut and burned herself many times.

Martha was married to Sam for two stormy years. She tricked him into marrying her by saying she was pregnant; then he discovered she was not pregnant. Martha idealized Sam as being "perfect," only to later berate him for being totally "bad." Every time Sam attempted to leave Martha, she would tell him he was the perfect man for her and threaten to kill herself. Once, when Martha was hospitalized, Sam divorced her and married someone else.

Today, Martha overdosed on sleeping pills again. Even though they have been divorced for three years, she immediately called Sam to tell him what she had done. Sam called emergency medical services (EMS) and headed for the emergency department of the hospital where Martha would be taken. After treatment in the emergency department, Martha was transferred to a bed on the medical unit.

Case Study

The primary nurse reviews Martha's chart after getting a preliminary report from the emergency department nurse. As the nurse approaches the client's room, she finds the ex-husband just leaving. He explains that his wife and two small children will be wondering why he isn't home. Martha yells out as he is leaving, "You are the only one who has ever cared about me." The ex-husband takes the nurse down the hall, out of Martha's hearing range, and tells the nurse how Martha always calls him to rescue her after overdosing and how she keeps trying to hold onto the relationship.

The nurse enters the room, introduces herself, and does a brief assessment. She notices that Martha has some scratches and burn marks on her arms. Martha talks about being lonely, bored, and feeling empty, as if she has no identity. She shares that she dropped out of college just one course before graduation and has had several jobs that lasted about six months each.

At the end of the shift, Martha tells the primary nurse that she is a "good nurse," and the only nurse on the unit who understands her. Martha shares that the other nurses don't care and that one nurse in particular has been mean to her.

The psychiatrist learns about the good nurses and bad nurses from Martha and decides to talk with the head nurse about the situation. The psychiatrist orders Martha to be placed under close observation consisting of checks every fifteen minutes. He asks the head nurse to arrange some in-service training for staff on caring for clients with BPD.

The next morning, as the primary nurse is looking for a brush for Martha's hair, she finds a collection of soda can pull-tabs. The nurse tells Martha she cannot have the pull-tabs and confiscates them. Martha becomes intensely angry, demanding that the primary nurse leave. Martha calls the gift shop and orders a rose for each of the "good nurses" but not for the "bad nurses." She provides the unit secretary a list of who is to get a rose.

Questions

1. What behaviors does Martha exhibit that match the diagnostic criteria for BPD?

2. Why does Martha tell the primary nurse she is the only nurse who understands her? Why does she advise the psychiatrist about the good nurses and the bad nurses?

3. What would you tell Martha when she says you are the only nurse who understands her and all the others are mean?

4. If you were delegated responsibility for planning in-service training on BPD, what critical content would you select and who would you ask to present?

5. What explanatory theories exist for why clients with BPD engage in splitting and self-mutilation?

6. If you were the primary nurse, how would you handle Martha's anger at having her pull-tabs confiscated? What should you do when you feel uncomfortable dealing with a client's anger?

7. What is the prognosis for clients with BPD? What treatment modalities are available? Do programs exist for the families of clients with BPD?

8. What nursing diagnoses would you write for this client? What interventions would your recommend for the top-priority nursing diagnosis?

9. What therapeutic interventions would you recommend for Martha's complaints of loneliness and boredom?

10. Do you think the primary nurse will receive one of the roses for the "good nurses"? What is the meaning of these roses? How should the primary nurse respond?

11. What team decisions, rules, or actions would be helpful to a primary nurse working with Martha?

Questions and Suggested Answers

1.   What behaviors does Martha exhibit that match the diagnostic criteria for BPD? The *Diagnostic and Statistical Manual of Mental Disorders* (APA, 2000) lists nine diagnostic criteria for BPD. A person must exhibit five of nine criteria to be diagnosed with BPD.

> **1.** Extreme efforts to hold onto relationships and avoid real or imagined abandonment (Martha tries to hold onto Sam. First, she falsely claimed she was pregnant so he would marry her. Now, after their divorce, she periodically calls him after overdosing.)

2. A pattern of intense, unstable interpersonal relationships that alternate between idealization and devaluation (At first, Martha sees the primary nurse as a good nurse, but she becomes a bad nurse when she takes away the soda can pull-tabs.)

3. Identity disturbance with a persistently unstable sense of self (Martha tells the nurse she feels she has no identity.)

4. Recurrent suicidal gestures or threats, or self-mutilating behavior (Martha has cut herself, burned herself, and taken overdoses of medication several times.)

5. Chronic feelings of emptiness (Martha talks often of being lonely and bored.)

6. Anger that is inappropriate and intense, or problems controlling anger (Martha displayed extreme anger with the primary nurse.)

7. Mood instability, with mood changes lasting a few hours or a few days

8. Transient, stress-related severe dissociative behaviors or paranoid ideation.

9. Impulsivity in two or more areas that are potentially self-destructive such as gambling, sex, spending, abusing drugs, binge eating, or driving recklessly.

While Martha needs to be further assessed in regard to the last three criteria, she appears to meet six of the nine criteria. Only five are required for the BPD diagnosis. Staff nurses do not diagnose BPD but can describe client's behavior that matches, or does not match, criteria.

Many clients with a diagnosis of BPD engage in self-mutilating behaviors such as burning themselves with the lit end of a cigarette or cutting or scratching themselves with a razor blade or a soda can pull-tab. More rarely, a client with BDP will engage in strangulating-type behaviors using bed linens or other means.

2. Why does Martha tell the primary nurse she is the only nurse who understands her? Why does she advise the psychiatrist about the good nurses and the bad nurses? When Martha tells the primary nurse that she is the only one who understands her and that the other nurses are mean to her, Martha is "splitting." *Splitting* is a defense mechanism whereby the person is not able to see both good and bad qualities in self and others, thus viewing self and others as all good or all bad. Splitting defends the person against the pain and hurt associated with real or perceived threats of rejection or abandonment. Martha is splitting when she tells the psychiatrist about the good nurses and the bad nurses. Staff members often use the term "splitting" to mean that the client is attempting to get the staff to fight among themselves by manipulating a "good" staff member or members to deal with another staff member or members on the client's bad list.

3. What would you tell Martha when she says you are the only nurse who understands her and all the others are mean? When a client says something like this, you can ignore the remark and change the subject. You also can respond by saying, "Yes, I do care about your well-being" or "You have helped me understand what is going on with you" and then changing the subject without going into what other nurses have said or done.

It is therapeutic to tell the client that if she has a problem with another nurse, she must discuss it and work it out with that person. If the complaint deals with possible abuse or neglect, you can discuss the matter with your supervisor, who will likely ask the client to put the complaint in writing. Depending on the situation, the client might be asked to sit down with the nurse being accused of abuse or neglect and discuss the matter in the supervisor's presence.

4. If you were delegated responsibility for planning in-service training on BPD, what critical content would you select and who would you ask to present? You could arrange for an experienced psychiatric nurse clinician to provide the staff information about BPD. If a psychiatric nurse clinician is not available, then a knowledgeable psychiatrist or psychologist could be asked. You should cover topics such as the behaviors seen in BPD and the traits that Martha manifests. You also should discuss splitting and manipulation, and how to deal with them therapeutically and professionally.

The staff should be advised that approximately 10 percent of clients with BPD do sooner or later commit suicide (Paris, 2005). This understanding is key, as many suicide attempts by clients with BPD might seem like gestures to get attention, hold on to people, or relieve feelings of emptiness or worthlessness.

5. What explanatory theories exist for why clients with BPD engage in splitting and self-mutilation? About 75 percent of the clients with BPD are female; most have been the victims of physical and/or sexual abuse and early parental loss or separation (APA, 2000; McLean and Gallop, 2003). One theory about splitting suggests that it somehow arises from the dissociation defense mechanism used by children who are experiencing sexual abuse. Just as dissociating spares children from the pain and feelings associated with abuse, splitting spares clients the pain and feelings from abandonment or loss. Also, depersonalization might play a role in self-mutilization. *Depersonalization* is the client's feeling of being outside of her body and looking at it. From this detached position, no pain is felt. Clients with BPD might dissociate or depersonalize when they feel abandoned, rejected, abused, or feel the pressure of increased responsibility. Clinicians need to assess and monitor a client with BPD for any self-mutilating ideas or behavior if any of these situations occurs. Clients often talk about self-mutilating acts, such as cutting themselves with coke tabs or razor blades or burning themselves with cigarettes, as ways to reaffirm that they are alive.

6. If you were the primary nurse, how would you handle Martha's anger at having her pull-tabs confiscated? What should you do when you feel uncomfortable dealing with a client's anger? It is therapeutic to recognize Martha's feelings by saying something like, "You seem very angry and upset about having your pull-tabs confiscated. It must be very difficult to know that you won't be able to hurt yourself when you want to do so. When you are ready, we can talk about these feelings and behaviors." It is important to stay calm and use a calm voice.

If you feel uncomfortable dealing with the client's anger, you should follow the same approach. However, you should then discuss your issues with anger with your supervisor and learn how to get help.

7. What is the prognosis for clients with BPD? What treatment modalities are available? Do programs exist for the families of clients with BPD? Nehls (2000) suggests that recovery is possible for clients with BPD. She recommends working on client-centered goals to achieve that goal. Likewise, research by Zanarini and associates (2003) found that the prognosis for clients with a diagnosis of BPD is better than previously recognized. Paris (2005) advises that compared to most other personality disorders—Schizophrenia or Bipolar Disorder—the prognosis for BPD is much better. According to Paris, 90 percent of the subjects with BPD in a long-term follow-up study who were diagnosed in their 20s no longer met the criteria for BPD by middle age and had notably improved functioning.

Lively (2005) points out that there is good reason why many people view BPD as difficult to treat. Clients with this personality disorder frequently have trouble engaging in treatment and when they do engage in treatment within the health care system, some deteriorate instead of improve. He also views BPD as a chronic disorder. Thus, he suggests keeping clients out of the hospital as much as possible and treating them on an outpatient basis. Lively also recommends identifying the client's assets and using them to develop relevant skills. He discusses several treatment modalities including Dialectical Behavior Therapy (DBT), Schema Therapy, Mentalization-Based Therapy, and pharmacotherapy such as fluvoxamine (Luvox), which decreases anger, impulsivity, and rapid mood shifts, and fluoxetine (Prozac), which decreases anger, depression, and impulsive aggression. Lively emphasizes that antidepressants take the edge off of BPD, but they never produce a remission of the disease. He underscores the need for new medications to treat personality disorders.

Lively (2005) describes DBT as an adaptation of Cognitive Behavioral Therapy that contains an eclectic mix of the effective methods found in several other therapies. DBT techniques target the client's mood instability and address impulsive behaviors. DBT applies behavioral analysis to incidents leading to self-injury and overdose, while emphasizing empathic responses to the client's distress. In so doing, the professional validates the client's feelings. The drawbacks to DBT are its intensiveness and expense (e.g., the initial phase takes one year).

Schema Therapy focuses on maladaptive schema resulting from adverse childhood experiences. Mentation-Based Therapy advances the idea that clients with BPD will benefit from mentalizing. "Essentially, mentalizing involves the capacity of individuals accurately to perceive, anticipate, and act on both their own mental states and the mental states of other people. One aspect of mentalizing involves the client feeling his own feelings, then imagining he is standing outside, which involves the person himself to accurately observe his own emotions (Twemlow, Fonagy, and Sacco, 2005, 1).

Lively (2005) describes the importance of communicating hope, conveying understanding and acceptance of the client's problems, and supporting treatment goals. He emphasizes the need to build a collaborative relationship with clients and maintain a consistent, validating treatment process. These approaches will help clients gain insight into how repeated patterns of action and past experiences contribute to their problems. He suggests not trying to change traits such as social withdrawal, mood shifting, and seeking sensation radically, but rather assisting clients to find ways to adapt these characteristics and use them in an acceptable way.

Hoffman and associates (2005) describe a program for family members of clients with BPD. Trained family members of clients with BPD present this twelve-week, multi-family program, using a manual, to others who have a family member with BPD. It is modeled after Family to Family, a program created by NAMI.

8. What nursing diagnoses would you write for this client? What interventions would your recommend for the top-priority nursing diagnoses? Possible nursing diagnoses for this client include: Risk for suicide, Impaired social interaction, Risk for self-directed mutilation, Ineffective coping, Identity disturbance, Chronic low self-esteem, and Risk for loneliness. The priority diagnoses are Risk for suicide and Risk for self-directed mutilation.

Clients at risk for suicide must be assessed at least each shift for degree of intent and magnitude (i.e., whether it has increased or decreased). The primary nurse can ask Martha, "When you took the overdose of pills and called Sam, you might have wanted to die, but perhaps you hoped you'd be rescued from death. Do you think this is a possibility?" You are planting an idea, not as an expert, but as a collaborator with the client. The next idea the nurse can plant is to suggest that attempting suicide and calling for rescue is a dangerous practice. The nurse could ask, "Have you ever thought about what might happen if your rescuer doesn't arrive in time to save you?" The client can be asked to journal on this topic and share it with the nurse. While journaling is not effective for every client, it does help many clients with BPD with their self-harm and other issues.

9. What therapeutic intervention would you recommend for Martha's complaints of loneliness and boredom? You might encourage Martha to consider adopting an appropriate pet. Many clients with BPD often have stormy, difficult interpersonal relationships in which they see others as all good or all bad, overvalue or undervalue them, and exhibit rapid swings from one polar position to another. Having a pet gives the client a constant, nonthreatening relationship.

10. Do you think the primary nurse will receive one of the roses for the "good nurses"? What is the meaning of these roses? How should the primary nurse respond? The primary nurse will not receive a rose unless she works through the confiscation of the pull-tabs and other issues affecting the nurse–client relationship. The client has put the primary nurse into the category of "bad nurse" because she denied Martha something she wants: a means to cut herself. The nurse can remind Martha that she is committed to helping her stay safe from harm and from harming herself. The nurse also can help the client talk this issue through and/or journal about it. Sometimes, posing a question works better than telling. For example, you might ask, "Why do you suppose I took away your pull-tabs?" or "If you were the nurse and I was the client, what would you do if I cut myself with pull-tabs?"

Receiving or not receiving the rose involves the client's maladaptive defense mechanism of splitting. Putting the roses in a vase in the report or break room for all the staff to enjoy would defuse this situation.

11. What team decisions, rules, or actions would be helpful to a primary nurse working with Martha? Helpful team decisions, rules, and actions include limiting the number of staff who work with Martha and assigning one primary nurse as case manager. This tactic limits the opportunities for Martha to split or manipulate the staff and helps send Martha a clear message. It also increases the possibility of building a therapeutic relationship with her. In addition, staff members need to agree not to react to Martha's attempts to manipulate or split; instead, the team should derive an overall approach to deal with any problems. Staff members must devise and enforce rules to protect Martha. If any staff members bend the rules for a manipulative client, it could prove disastrous.

References

American Psychiatric Association (APA). (2000). *Diagnostic and Statistical Manual of Mental Disorders, 4th ed.* Text Revision. Washington, DC: APA.

Hoffman, J. et al. (2005). "Effectiveness of a Program for Relatives of Persons with Borderline Personality Disorder." *Family Process* 44: 217–225.

Lively, W. J. (2005). "Principles and Strategies for Treating Personality Disorders." *Canadian Journal of Psychiatry* 50(8): 442–451.

McLean, L. M. and R. Gallop. (2003). "Implications of Childhood Sexual Abuse for Adult Borderline Personality Disorder and Complex Posttraumatic Stress Disorder." *American Journal of Psychiatry* 160(2): 369–371.

Nehls, N. (2000). "Recovering: A Process of Empowerment." *Advances in Nursing Science* 22(4): 62–70.

Paris, J. (2005). "Recent Advances in the Treatment of Borderline Personality Disorder." *Canadian Journal of Psychiatry* 50(8): 435–441.

Twemlow, S. W., P. Fonagy, and F. C. Sacco (2005). "A Developmental Approach to Mentalizing Communities: I A Model for Social Change." *Menninger Bulletin* in progress available at http://www.freudconference.com/online_papers/Mentl_8_9_05_ST.htm. Assessed June 9, 2006.

Zanarini, M. C., et al. (2003). "The Longitudinal Course of Borderline Psychopathology: 6 Year Prospective Follow Up of the Phenomenology of Borderline Personality Disorder." *American Journal of Psychiatry* 160(2): 274–284.

Clark

GENDER

M

AGE

20

SETTING

- City jail

ETHNICITY

- White American

CULTURAL CONSIDERATIONS

PREEXISTING CONDITION

COEXISTING CONDITION

- Alcohol abuse
- Marijuana abuse

COMMUNICATION

DISABILITY

SOCIOECONOMIC

- Low income
- Raised in housing project

SPIRITUAL/RELIGIOUS

PHARMACOLOGIC

- Carbamazepine (Tegretol)

PSYCHOSOCIAL

LEGAL

- Incarcerated

ETHICAL

ALTERNATIVE THERAPY

- The nurse must avoid being manipulated by the client

PRIORITIZATION

DELEGATION

ANTISOCIAL PERSONALITY DISORDERS

Level of difficulty: High

Overview: Requires critical thinking, judgment, and therapeutic communication skills. The nurse must set limits and enforce rules in a nonpunitive, empathic manner. Also, the nurse must help the client gain insight into how his behavior affects others and teach him empathy so he can behave in a socially acceptable manner.

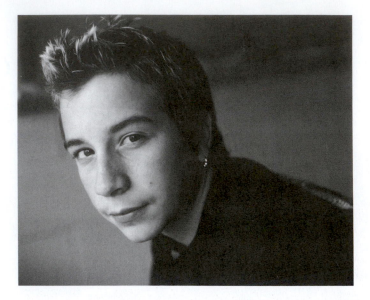

Client Profile

Clark is a 20-year-old white American male who was raised in the "poor section" of town. His father was rarely home and took no responsibility for either the children or the bills. When Clark's father did get a job, he either quit or was fired within a week. After doing time in prison, he died of alcoholism. Clark's mother works two jobs.

Clark has been in and out of trouble since he was 11 years old. His first incident involved drowning a neighbor's cat. Clark explained, "I was just seeing if the cat could swim." Subsequently, Clark was accused of damaging neighbors' property and stealing, Clark, who doesn't get along well with authority figures, broke all the rules when he was in school (e.g., skipping school to drink beer and smoke pot). He usually convinced his mother to take his side against the authorities. He talked his mother into other things, too (e.g., "borrowing" her brother's credit card and buying Clark expensive tennis shoes and a motorcycle without any thought of repayment).

When Clark was age 15, he was caught in a neighbor's home when the neighbor returned in the middle of the day. The neighbor called the police. Clark was sent to a residential treatment center for adolescents. He was diagnosed as having Conduct Disorder. After a six-week stay, he was released to his mother. Clark committed several burglaries at age 17 and was incarcerated. He used his one phone call to reach Trisha; a former classmate; Clark convinced her of his innocence. Trisha borrowed money from her mother and put up bail. Later, Clark served a short sentence and was released on probation.

Clark talked Trisha into leaving her parents, getting a job and an apartment, and marrying him. Clark tried several jobs but always had a good reason for leaving them. He scared his wife by driving recklessly and verbally threatening people in bars. He got a couple of speeding tickets and frequently wrote bad checks to pay them. Over a twelve-month period, Clark lied to his wife about looking for work, ran up her credit card, disappeared with her car, and had affairs with other women. He used her credit card to pay for the hotel. Trisha was stuck with the credit card debt and a car payment for a car she no longer possessed. She decided to divorce Clark. She characterized him as indifferent and uncaring about hurting or mistreating others. She could not recall Clark ever saying he was sorry for anything.

Case Study

Clark is in jail for scamming an elderly couple out of their money. As the jail's evening nurse makes her rounds, she stops to see if Clark has any health problems. He tells her, "You're too pretty to be a nurse. You should be a model." He engages the nurse in conversation and then asks, "If you would make a phone call for me, I'd give you $60. It's just between us. Don't tell anyone about this."

The nurse schedules Clark for a visit with the psychiatrist who comes daily to the jail. After examining Clark and getting a history, the psychiatrist writes a diagnosis of Antisocial Personality Disorder (APD). He adds Alcohol Abuse and Marijuana Abuse. Clark has a pending driving while intoxicated (DWI) charge, and his drug screen is positive for marijuana. The psychiatrist writes an order for carbamazepine (Tegretol XR), with vital signs taken every shift.

Questions

1. If you were the nurse, how would you respond to Clark's comments about your looks and his proposition regarding the phone call?

2. What is the essential feature of APD? Does this client demonstrate this feature?

3. What criteria must the client meet to qualify for a diagnosis of APD? Does this client's history support this diagnosis?

4. Why did the psychiatrist prescribe carbamazepine? What do you need to know about carbamazepine? What do you need to teach the client about carbamazepine?

5. Are males or females more likely to be diagnosed with APD? What is the prevalence of APD?

6. Does APD run in families? Is there any evidence that Clark's father might have had APD? What causes APD?

Questions (continued)

7. Do all criminals have APD, and are they treated for this disorder? Are clients with APD commonly found in other settings?

8. What role could Clark's culture of poverty and drug abuse play in the development of his symptoms or his response to treatment?

9. Do clients with APD get better or is it impossible to change antisocial personality traits?

10. What nursing diagnoses would you likely write for Clark?

11. What nursing interventions would you likely implement for these nursing diagnoses?

12. What current treatment modalities could be used with Clark?

Questions and Suggested Answers

1.   If you were the nurse, how would you respond to Clark's comments about your looks and his proposition regarding the phone call? Whenever a client focuses on you, either being complimentary or seeking personal information, you need to refocus the attention on the client, especially when that client is diagnosed with APD. He will try to establish a special relationship to get what he wants, without any regard for you or anyone else. It is not therapeutic to perpetuate this behavior. Your professional role is to help the client with medical and psychological problems, not to have your ego needs met. You must not accept money from the client. In addition, you must deal with the client's attempt to abuse a telephone rule of the jail. You must be familiar with the rules and enforce them consistently. The client with APD has little or no concern for rules. You can encourage Clark to discuss his motives for wanting to have you make a phone call for him, but he must be held to the rules of the jail. You can be empathic, but you need to state the rules in a clear, nonpunitive manner. If he does have good reason for having a call made for him, you must present it to your peers and supervisor so a joint decision can be made.

2.   What is the essential feature of APD? Does this client demonstrate this feature? The essential feature of APD is a pervasive pattern of disregard for others' rights that starts in childhood or early adolescence and remains in adulthood. Clark has a long history of taking things from others, destroying their property, and buying things on others' credit cards with no thought of paying them back. Clark left his ex-wife in debt created by his adultery. He scammed some elderly people out of money. These behaviors seem to verify a lack of regard for the rights of others.

3. What criteria must the client meet to qualify for a diagnosis of APD? Does this client's history support this diagnosis? The following criteria must be met to make this diagnosis:

- Having three or more of seven behavioral patterns indicating a pervasive pattern of disregarding and violating the rights of others:
  1. Not conforming to social norms, doing things that are grounds for arrest (Clark has driven recklessly while intoxicated and has a pending charge of DWI. He has written checks with no funds and threatened others in bars. He has scammed an elderly couple, leading to an arrest and incarceration.)
  2. Being deceitful as evidenced by lying repeatedly, using aliases, or conning other people for fun or personal gain (Clark lied repeatedly to his wife about looking for work and conned her out of her credit card and her car. He also conned an elderly couple. He is trying to con the nurse in the jail into breaking the rules.)
  3. Being impulsive or not planning ahead (There is no evidence that this client plans ahead.)
  4. Being irritable or aggressive, as evidenced by a number of physical fights or assaults (Clark has gotten into arguments in bars, which is not quite physical fights or assaults, but still demonstrates irritability and aggression.)
  5. Lacking regard for safety of self and/or others (Clark has driven recklessly.)
  6. Being consistently irresponsible, as evidenced by failure to have consistent good work behavior or to be responsible in financial obligations (Clark runs up bills rather than paying them. He has little work history.)
  7. Lacking remorse, as evidenced by indifference or rationalizing reasons for hurting, mistreating, or stealing from others (He was not mistreating the cat, just seeing if it could swim. Clark's wife says she has never known him to apologize.)
- Is at least 18 years old (Clark is 25.)
- Demonstrates symptoms of Conduct Disorder (CD) before age 15 (Clark exhibited a number of early symptoms of CD: aggression toward a neighbor's cat, breaking and entering, stealing, truancy from school, and conning others. Clark actually was diagnosed with CD, although a diagnosis of CD is not a prerequisite to a diagnosis of APD.) The person need only have a history of the symptoms of CD.
- Antisocial behavior is not exclusively during a Manic Episode or due to Schizophrenia (Clark has no evidence of having Bipolar Disorder or Schizophrenia.)

4. Why did the psychiatrist prescribe carbamazepine? What do you need to know about carbamazepine? What do you need to teach the client about carbamazepine? Carbamazepine is an anticonvulsant medication that is used to prevent seizures. It also is used to target and lessen the impulsivity associated with CD, APD, and other disorders. It is thought to prevent the seizures associated with alcohol withdrawal when a client is sufficiently dependent on alcohol to be at risk for seizures. The nurse must ensure periodic complete blood cell (CBC) counts are performed.

You need to teach the client that carbamazepine is to be taken as ordered, not to skip doses, and to discuss discontinuing the medication with the health care provider before tapering off and discontinuing it. Advise the client that the coating of extended-release versions is not absorbed, but rather is passed through the feces; thus, the client might see the coating in the stool. Teach the client not to take alcohol with this medication, to wear sunglasses and use sunscreen to prevent photosensitivity, and to use chewing gum or mouthwash to relieve dry mouth. Instruct the client to notify health care professionals that he is taking carbamazepine before undergoing any medical or surgical procedures.

5. Are males or females more likely to be diagnosed with APD? What is the prevalence of APD? In the general population, prevalence is approximately 1 percent for females and 3 percent for males. Higher rates, still predominantly male, are reported in various treatment settings. The highest prevalence rates occur in substance abuse treatment programs and prisons (APA, 2000). Pajer and associates (2001), noticing that the incidence of aggressive and antisocial behaviors among female adolescents seemed to be on the rise, compared early morning plasma cortisol levels in forty-seven adolescent girls, some of whom had Conduct Disorder (and no other identified psychiatric problems) and some of whom did not. The girls with antisocial behaviors had significantly lower morning plasma cortisol levels. This research indicates that girls with antisocial behaviors have some biochemical difference from girls who do not have antisocial behaviors.

6. Does APD run in families? Is there any evidence that Clark's father might have had APD? What causes APD? Clark's father did not keep a job for long, and he was irresponsible in regard to the bills and the children. He spent time in prison and died of alcoholism. Thus, Clark's father appears to have some traits of APD. Having an antisocial or alcoholic parent increases the risk of a person developing APD (Dilley, 2004).

Frisch and Frisch (2006, 375) cite remarks from Fox Butterfield's 1994 book entitled *All God's Children: The Basket Family and the American Tradition of Violence* wherein Butterfield describes a "single remarkably violent family in which the disorder can be traced back as far as 1820."

While genetics no doubt plays a role in the cause of APD, the actual cause(s) of APD and other personality disorders remains unknown. Evidence points to many causative factors, including genetics and environment. Bassarath (2001, 728) suggests that "abnormal prefrontal (and probably subcortical) circuitry are very likely involved in antisocial behaviour." Even with this evidence of abnormal structure and function in people with APD, Bassarath advises against attributing cause to either nature or nurture, given the links between the brain, environment, and behavior.

Ward (2004, 1505) suggests that the various symptom complexes specific to each personality disorders "are caused by a combination of hereditary temperamental traits and environmental and developmental events. The relative percentage of these genetic and environmental factors vary with each specific disorder."

7. Do all criminals have APD, and are they treated for this disorder? Are clients with APD commonly found in other settings? Not all criminals have APD. Fazel and Danesh (2002) found that prisoners were several times more likely to have psychoses and major depression than APD. Some 65 percent of the prisoners they studied had some sort of personality disorder, with only 21 percent having APD. However, prisoners were still "ten times more likely to have antisocial personality disorder than the general population" (Fazel and Danesh, 2002, 545). Fazel and Danesh expressed concern that with several million prisoners worldwide believed to have serious mental disorders, there is little known about how well prison services are addressing this problem.

Ward (2004, 1505) says that clients with "personality disorders (including APD) are common in primary care settings" and that the psychosocial functioning of these clients can vary widely. Not all clients with APD or traits of APD are found in jails or prison. Some hide their pathology well or escape the law through luck or other means. Some even find their way to important positions in companies and public service.

8. What role could Clark's culture of poverty and drug abuse play in the development of his symptoms or his response to treatment? Kirkman (2002) cites an article by Mitchell and Blair who suggest that, while a biological predisposition determines whether people have emotional difficulties associated with the psychopathology of this disorder, it is the adverse social environment that provides the conditions necessary to develop the behaviors associated with the disorder. If Clark had been born into a family with social advantage and affluence; if his parents had held strong social consciences and modeled ethical behaviors; and if neither he nor his parents had abused alcohol or other drugs, then his personality would have been different. The question remains, however, about whether or not he would have still met the criteria for APD but with a different pattern and string of specific behaviors. Not everyone who comes from a similar background as Clark's has APD. Perhaps, there are positive and negative factors that pull against each other and determine whether a person's behaviors fall inside or outside the criterion for APD as provided by the *Diagnostic and Statistical Manual of Mental Disorders* (APA, 2000).

9. Do clients with APD get better or is it impossible to change antisocial personality traits? The *Diagnostic and Statistical Manual of Mental Disorders* (APA, 2000) describes a decline in symptom severity by the fourth decade of life in clients diagnosed with APD. Clients who reach age 40 tend not to be engaged in criminal behavior and experience a significant decrease in other antisocial behaviors and substance use. Seivewright and associates (2002) found that clients who had APD and Histrionic Personality Disorder had significantly less pronounced traits at the end of their twelve-year study.

10. What nursing diagnoses would you likely write for Clark? Nursing diagnoses might include:

- Impaired social interaction
- Ineffective coping
- Ineffective denial
- Noncompliance
- Risk for other-directed violence

11. What nursing interventions would you likely implement for these nursing diagnoses?

- Establish firm limits with all staff, ensuring consistent application of rules to enhance feelings of client security and reduce attempts to "conn" and manipulate the staff
- Stress positive consequences for good behavior, and discuss and implement negative consequences consistently
- Have staff share with client how his antisocial behaviors make them feel right after the client exhibits the behavior
- Encourage significant others and peers to share with client how his behavior makes them feel
- Accept client but not his antisocial behaviors; explain the difference to him
- Offer recreational and occupational skills training

12. What current treatment modalities could be used with Clark? Some treatment facilities, such as adolescent treatment centers, alcohol and drug abuse treatment centers, and prisons, use psychodrama with clients with APD. At different times, the client plays the role of victim and aggressor in order to develop the capacity for empathy and remorse. Nurses at any level can seek training in psychodrama. Depending on their level of training and ability, nurses can serve as leaders, coleaders, or play roles as part of the group. Only trained lay therapists should use psychodrama.

Prisons also have clients meet and talk with victims as another means of increasing empathy and remorse for hurtful acts. Prisoners are sometimes given the chance to make amends with the victim.

Medication is not a treatment of choice. Current medications do not target the antisocial behaviors, although impulsiveness often responds to carbamazepine. Other medications can treat the symptoms of depression, if present.

Mayer (2001) looked at the effects of punishment and consequences (rather than positive reward systems) in schools on dropout rate and aggressive and antisocial behaviors. He found a relationship and suggests that a punitive environment helps move children with aggressive and antisocial behaviors toward the symptoms and diagnosis of APD. He recommends positive reward systems for both school administrators and parents to help prevent dropout and antisocial behavior. Some treatment programs use positive reward systems along with consequences to work with clients who have APD. In a token or point-system economy, positive behavior helps the client earn privileges and desired items.

Clients with APD benefit from occupational and leisure skills training as well as communication and relationship skills training.

References

American Psychiatric Association (APA). (2000) *Diagnostic and Statistical Manual of Mental Disorders, 4th ed.* Text Revision. Washington, DC: APA.

Bassarath, L. (2001). "Neuroimaging Studies of Antisocial Behavior." *Canadian Journal of Psychiatry* 46(8): 728–733.

Dilley, J. W. (2004). "Antisocial Personality Disorder" in *MedlinePlus Medical Encyclopedia*. Available online at http://www.nlm.nih.gov/medlineplus/ency/article/000921.htm.

Fazel, S. and J. Danesh. (2002). "Serious Mental Disorder in 23,000 Prisoners: A Systemic Review of 62 Surveys." *Lancet* 359(9306): 545–551.

Frisch, N. C. and L. E. Frisch. (2006). *Psychiatric Mental Health Nursing, 3d ed.* Albany, NY: Thomson Delmar Learning.

Kirkman, C. A. (2002). "Non-Incarcerated Psychopaths: Why We Need to Know More About the Psychopaths That Live Among Us." *Journal of Psychiatric and Mental Health Nursing* 9(2): 155–160.

Mayer, G. R. (2001). "Antisocial Behavior: Its Causes and Prevention Within Our Schools." *Education and Treatment of Children* 24(4): 414–430.

Pajer, K., et al. (2001). "Decreased Cortisol Levels in Adolescent Girls with Conduct Disorder." *Archives of General Psychiatry* 58(3): 297–302.

Seivewright, H., et al. (2002). "Change in Personality Status in Neurotic Disorders." *Lancet* 359 (9325): 2253–2255.

Ward, R. K. (2004). "Assessment and Management of Personality Disorders." *American Family Physician* 70(8): 1505–1512.

CASE STUDY 3

Ralph

GENDER

M

AGE

37

SETTING

- Rehabilitation hospital

ETHNICITY

- Mexican American

CULTURAL CONSIDERATIONS

- Hispanic

PREEXISTING CONDITION

COEXISTING CONDITION

- Hip fracture

COMMUNICATION

DISABILITY

SOCIOECONOMIC

- Inherited large sum of money and property

SPIRITUAL/RELIGIOUS

PHARMACOLOGIC

PSYCHOSOCIAL

- Bizarre behavior distances people
- Comes close to people then distances

LEGAL

- Humane society cruelty charges
- Property condemnation proceedings
- Right to sign out of hospital against medical advice (AMA)

ETHICAL

ALTERNATIVE THERAPY

- Herbs used by *curanderos*

PRIORITIZATION

DELEGATION

PERSONALITY DISORDERS: SCHIZOTYPAL PERSONALITY DISORDER

Level of difficulty: High

Overview: Requires the nurse to use critical thinking to select effective approaches to help a client who is not comfortable around others. The nurse must convey liking the person, but not always the person's behavior. The nurse needs to become familiar with the client's culture and help the client return to cultural practices that are therapeutic.

Client Profile

Ralph is a 37-year-old male who is often described as "odd" or "eccentric." His brother, Robert, characterizes Ralph as distant and unemotional; he recalls Ralph laughing in an odd way when a family pet died. When questioned about this, Ralph replied, "I sensed the dog would die." Robert relates that Ralph has acquaintances, but no close friends. The acquaintances are fellow stargazers who are "kind of odd and different themselves," according to the brother. Robert says, "Ralph claims he can predict plays a local soccer team will make. Ralph says he is responsible for the team winning or losing by watching or not watching the game."

Ralph had a job as a night watchman at a factory. Ralph avoided contact with other nightshift employees, fearing they would say bad things about him and get him fired. He also avoided contact with his boss whenever he could.

Ralph stopped working when his grandfather died and left him $10 million, a cattle ranch, and a city office building fully leased to professional people. Ralph didn't feed the cattle, saying God intended them to eat grass. The humane society charged him with cruelty to animals when a neighbor reported the cattle were starving. Ralph failed to renew contracts with the tenants of his office building. He would run in and out of their offices for brief periods, sometimes saying things the tenants thought were bizarre. He did not maintain the building. Eventually, all the tenants left and the building's condition deteriorated. The city condemned it and plans to sell it for back taxes.

Years ago, Ralph invited a girl to meet him at a high-school dance. When she arrived, Ralph said a few words to her and then disappeared for a half hour. He returned for five minutes and then left again. He repeated this process until the girl, thinking Ralph was "extremely weird," left without telling Ralph goodbye.

Recently, a woman and her child moved in with Ralph. He is unsure how this came about. She describes life with Ralph as "bizarre," saying Ralph will not spend any money if he can help it. He does not use the electric lights as this "energy could run through (his) body in a dangerous way." She relates, "Ralph told me he can read my mind and his grandmother's mind, even though his grandmother lives some distance away."

Case Study

Ralph is being admitted to a rehabilitation hospital to recover from a broken hip sustained from falling off a horse. His family health care provider interviews Ralph's brother and grandmother, who accompanied Ralph to the hospital, and includes information about his psychosocial behavior in his history and physical. The health care provider notes in the chart that the client's behavior is consistent with traits of Schizotypal Personality Disorder.

The nurse doing the admission assessment notices that Ralph's affect is constricted, and he seems wary when talking to her about treatment plans. Ralph asks her to leave after a few minutes. The nurse says, "I have some tasks to do. I will come back in about thirty minutes. If you need something, call me." Ralph puts the call light on five minutes later and asks the nurse to get him several herbs, as he is a *curandero*. He claims he can heal himself and won't need to bother any physical therapists, occupational therapists, or other staff members. He thinks he will be able to go home in a couple of days. The nurse considers how best to respond.

Later, the nurse enters Ralph's room to give him some medication and finds fourteen extended family members with him. Ralph says he will be glad when visiting hours are over. Then, in Spanish, he tells his visitors to go to the cafeteria while he talks to the nurse. When Ralph is alone with the nurse, he asks the nurse to do something to stop so many visitors from coming to see him. He only wants his brother and grandmother to visit.

Questions

1. Ralph's health care provider charts a note suggesting a diagnosis of Schizotypal Personality Disorder. Do you agree with the health care provider's assessment? If so, why Schizotypal Personality Disorder rather than Schizoid Personality Disorder?

2. The admitting nurse leaves Ralph alone for thirty minutes even though he seems anxious. Why would the nurse leave him? What other choice could the nurse have made?

3. Ralph claims to be a *curandero*. What is a *curandero*?

4. What therapeutic response could the nurse offer when Ralph says he is a *curandero* and can cure himself? What additional actions should the nurse take regarding Ralph's statement that he will leave the hospital in two days.

5. Why would fourteen members of Ralph's extended family visit him? If you were the nurse, how would you deal with Ralph's request to stop their visits?

6. If you were the nurse, what psychosocial assessment(s) would you do? What nursing diagnoses would you most likely write for Ralph?

7. What nursing interventions would most be most helpful?

8. What would happen if Ralph decides to leave the hospital after two days and the family objects?

9. What treatment modalities are being used with clients who have Schizotypal Personality Disorder?

10. Is there a familial pattern with Schizotypal Personality Disorder? What causes Schizotypal Personality Disorder?

11. What is the course of Schizotypal Personality Disorder?

Questions and Suggested Answers

1. Ralph's health care provider charts a note suggesting a diagnosis of Schizotypal Personality Disorder. Do you agree with the health care provider's assessment? If so, why Schizotypal Personality Disorder rather than Schizoid Personality Disorder? If you compare the client's behavior with the behavioral traits found in the diagnostic criteria for each disorder (see the table below), you will find that Ralph's behavior best matches Schizotypal Personality Disorder. He exhibits suspiciousness, ideas of reference, and odd or magical thinking consistent with Schizotypal Personality Disorder, but not present in Schizoid Personality Disorder.

Schizoid Personality Disorder Behaviors	Client's Behavior	Schizotypal Personality Disorder Behaviors	Client's Behavior
Pervasive pattern of movement away from social relationships with limited range of emotional expression in interpersonal settings starting by young adult age and seen in different contexts with four or more of the following behaviors:	Has movement away from social relationships, but periodically and briefly moves toward relationships Has a limited range of expressions (Also look at the four behaviors)	Pervasive pattern of deficits in social and interpersonal relationships, discomfort with close relationships Eccentric behavior and thought distortions reduce capacity for friendships with five of the following behaviors:	Has deficits in social and interpersonal relationships, discomfort with close relationships Definitely has eccentric behavior, thought distortions, reduced capacity for friendships (Also look at the five behaviors)
1. Does not want or enjoy close relationships, including those related to being a member of a family	Might want close relationships but not able to manage them Does relate to immediate family	1. Has ideas of reference	Yes, a team won or lost based on what he was thinking

(Continued)

Schizoid Personality Disorder Behaviors	Client's Behavior	Schizotypal Personality Disorder Behaviors	Client's Behavior
2. Chooses solitary activities most or all of the time	Yes	2. Has odd beliefs or magical thinking not consistent with cultural norms	Yes, thinks he is a *curandero* and can cure people Believes he can read minds
3. Little or no interest in having sex with another person	Possibly true, although he has made attempts to date and lives with a woman	3. Unusual perceptual experiences	Yes
4. Little or no pleasure in most or all activities	Does have some interests such as stargazing, hiking, and horseback riding	4. Has odd thinking and speech	
5. Seems indifferent to praise or criticism of others	No, he fears being criticized	5. Has suspicious or paranoid ideation	Yes, feared other employees would say bad things about him
6. Appears to have emotional coldness or flattened affect or detachment from others	Affect is constricted rather than flattened	6. Affect is inappropriate at times or constricted	Yes, he laughed when dog died Nurse notices constricted affect
		7. Has peculiar, odd, or eccentric behavior or appearance	Yes
7. Has no close friends or confidants except for first-degree relatives	Yes	8. No close friends or confidants except for first-degree relatives	Yes

(Continued)

Schizoid Personality Disorder Behaviors	Client's Behavior	Schizotypal Personality Disorder Behaviors	Client's Behavior
		9. Social anxiety that is paranoid in nature, excessive, and doesn't improve with familiarity	Yes

Adapted from *Diagnostic and Statistical Manual of Mental Disorders* (APA, 2000).

2. The admitting nurse leaves Ralph alone for thirty minutes even though he seems anxious. Why would the nurse leave him? What other choice could the nurse have made? The nurse leaves Ralph alone so he can have time to reduce his anxiety, which escalates when he is around people for longer periods of time. The nurse is trying to build a level of trust with the client. One technique used with new clients is to make the first meeting brief, leave, and return shortly. The client often responds better on the second contact, as the nurse now seems familiar. Another technique for building trust is to tell a client you will return in a certain period of time and then ensure you arrive back on time. By demonstrating an ability to keep your word, you can build trust in clients, especially in those who are suspicious of others.

Alternatively, the nurse could have distracted Ralph by giving him a task to do, such as unpacking his belongings. She also could have adopted a quiet, calm approach and kept the interaction focused on nonthreatening topics, easing questions into the conversation rather than coming across as an authoritative interrogator.

3. Ralph claims to be a *curandero*. What is a *curandero*? A *curandero* is a holistic folk healer, typically found in Hispanic cultures. The *curandero* uses herbs, rituals, prayers, diets, cleansings, and massage to bring about healing. Healing might focus on a health problem, or it could involve getting rid of a spell put on by another person. In the Hispanic culture, illness is often thought to be the result of a *mal ojo* or "evil eye" cast on a person. Illness also is sometimes attributed to envy or fright. For example, a mother being frightened during pregnancy could cause mental illness or physical illness in a child.

4. What therapeutic response could the nurse offer when Ralph says he is a *curandero* and can cure himself? What additional actions should the

nurse take regarding Ralph's statement that he will leave the hospital in two days? The nurse can ignore Ralph's initial statement and respond only to the second part. Ignoring his first statement avoids reinforcing his belief. There are at least three reasons not to confront the statement about being a *curandero* as false:

1. If it were odd or magical thinking and not reality, confronting the belief would only reinforce it.
2. Challenging the statement would not help build the nurse–client relationship.
3. Ralph might be a *curandero* or he might want to become one. Studying could prove helpful in connecting him with his culture.

Electing not to get into a discussion about *curanderos,* but to address the second part of his statement (i.e., he will cure himself and leave in two days) recognizes the greater importance of working with Ralph to stay in rehabilitation until he is able to care for himself at home or finds someone he can trust to care for him adequately.

The nurse can reassure the client that he will be safe and well cared for in the rehabilitation hospital. The nurse also could distract the client into a conversation that helps the client move forward toward meeting goals. For example, the nurse could say, "Tell me one thing you need to accomplish in order to be able to take care of yourself at home."

The nurse must chart Ralph's statement, pass this information on in report, and advise the health care provider that Ralph has indicated he might leave in two days. The nurse must recognize that this client could decide to leave even sooner. He has the right to sign himself out. The health care provider has the choice to discharge him or inform him that he is leaving against medical advice (AMA). The nurse must be familiar with hospital policy regarding leaving AMA. Usually the client is asked to sign a form saying he realizes he is leaving AMA and chooses to do so. If he leaves without telling anyone and signing the AMA form, it is assumed that he left AMA. The AMA status helps protect the hospital and staff, including the nurse, in case of a lawsuit.

5. Why would fourteen members of Ralph's extended family visit him? If you were the nurse, how would you deal with Ralph's request to stop their visits? In the Hispanic culture, it is normal for the extended family to go with an ill family member to the hospital or visit the family member while there. As Ralph is Hispanic, this is the most likely explanation. Yet, Ralph's personality traits conflict with his cultural norms.

There are many acceptable ways to deal with Ralph's request to limit visitors. The nurse could ascertain which family member has the most influence over the others and talk with that person about getting the family to move to another room to visit with each other, allowing Ralph to rest. You might begin by telling this family member that you realize everyone has come a long way to be with Ralph, but he needs to rest. After the family has moved to another room, you might negotiate with Ralph as to whether he would agree to see the whole family together for just long enough to say goodbye or just one family member at a time for a quick goodbye. Short, brief visits might fit better with Ralph's history of dashing in and out (i.e., when talking to the girl at the dance or his tenants).

If Ralph still refuses to see his extended family, you must tactfully break this news to his family. Since some family members do not speak English, you should enlist the help of a native Spanish speaker who can not only help you with the translation, but also assist the family in understanding why they cannot visit with Ralph. Notably, Ralph's request runs counter to the customs of his culture and seems indicative of Schizotypal Personality Disorder.

6. If you were the nurse, what psychosocial assessment(s) would you do? What nursing diagnoses would you most likely write for Ralph? You need to find out more about this client's relationship with his family and who matters most to him. You also need to learn more about his relationship with the woman living in his home, especially his goals with respect to that relationship. You need to assess for sources of support and possible motivation for any behavioral changes regarding interpersonal relationships.

Probable nursing diagnoses for this client include:

- Altered thought processes
- Impaired social interaction
- Ineffective coping
- Anxiety

7. What nursing interventions would most be most helpful? The most helpful interventions would serve to build trust and maintain a trusting relationship between client and nurse first, and then help increase trust in others. The nurse should communicate unconditional acceptance for the client. The underlying personality should not be the focus of change. Behaviors that cause the client difficulty should be the focus of goals and interventions. For example, Ralph needs to learn social communication skills. One goal might be for Ralph to sit and talk (or stand and talk) for five minutes to one person rather than dashing in and dashing out. Behavior modification techniques employing positive reinforcement for behavior approximating the desired behavior would help Ralph meet this goal. When evaluating the nursing process, this goal, if met, could be revised to include not only talking for five minutes but staying on topic, or the time frame for interaction could be revised upward.

The nurse should encourage Ralph's connection with his culture. The nurse can communicate an interest in his culture and arrange to have foods, artwork, and other things from the Hispanic culture brought in.

The nurse also must teach Ralph, and anyone caring for him, about his medical care in preparation for discharge.

8. What would happen if Ralph decides to leave the hospital after two days and the family objects? If one of Ralph's family members feels strongly about him not leaving the rehabilitation hospital and believes he is not mentally competent to make decisions in his own best interest, this person could petition the court to be appointed his guardian. The family member would have to present evidence that Ralph is not competent to make his own decisions. Letting the cattle die and a building deteriorate could serve as evidence, as well as instances where Ralph made poor health decisions. The guardian could then attempt to have Ralph held in the rehabilitation hospital until he is ready to be discharged.

Many ethical issues surround this topic. Does the nurse think Ralph needs a legal guardian? Does the family know about guardianship? Should the nurse tell them about this option? The nurse needs to discuss these issues with a supervisor, Ralph's health care provider, and possibly the ethics committee of the hospital.

9. What treatment modalities are being used with clients who have Schizotypal Personality Disorder? Treatment commonly requires professional help with reality testing and sorting fantasy from reality. The person with Schizotypal Personality traits or diagnosed with Schizotypal Personality Disorder typically has distortion of reality, and it requires skill to know when and how to go about helping the client with reality testing. Treatment will include building an alliance with the client and working on developing a trusting relationship.

Supportive group experiences are generally part of treatment, if possible. Medication is not currently a standard part of treatment. If, however, a client has brief periods of psychosis under stress, then antipsychotics could be prescribed.

10. Is there a familial pattern with Schizotypal Personality Disorder? What causes Schizotypal Personality Disorder? In some cases, a client with Schizotypal Personality Disorder will have a family member with similar traits or with a diagnosis of Schizophrenia or Schizoid Personality Disorder. This finding suggests an increased prevalence of Schizotypal Personality Disorder in families with Schizophrenia and Schizoid Personality Disorder.

Research is under way exploring the biologic relationship between Schizotypal Personality Disorder and Schizophrenia. In addition, Schizotypal Personality Disorder could have similar causes to those of Schizophrenia.

Dickey and associates (1999) found a less-than-usual amount of left superior temple gyrus (STG) gray matter volume in subjects with Schizotypal Personality Disorder. Farmer and coworkers (2000) explored the differences between subjects with Schizotypal Personality Disorder and persons with Schizophrenia. They found that subjects with Schizotypal Personality Disorder have more intact visual perception than those with Schizophrenia. In addition, subjects with Schizotypal Personality Disorder exhibited memory deficits.

A *Brown University Child and Adolescent Behavior Letter* (2000) presents research findings that support the idea that Schizotypal Personality Disorder is related to "prenatal neurodevelopmental problems."

Researchers have also studied hair whorls, cortisol release, and a variety of physical factors for any connection to Schizotypal Personality Disorders.

11. What is the course of Schizotypal Personality Disorder? The course of Schizotypal Personality Disorder is chronic. While the behavioral traits of some personality disorders diminish as the client reaches a certain decade of life (e.g., Antisocial Personality Disorder), the traits of Schizotypal Personality Disorder are not expected to change much. This does not mean that the health care team cannot work with this client and help him modify some behaviors or take on new behaviors to replace especially troublesome ones. The nurse also can work with the family to help them gain insight into the client's behavior and needs, and how to best support him. A small percentage of people with Schizotypal Personality Disorder are eventually diagnosed with Schizophrenia or some other psychotic disorder (APA, 2000).

References

American Psychiatric Association (APA). (2000). *Diagnostic and Statistical Manual of Mental Disorders, 4th ed.* Text Revision. Washington, DC: APA.

Dickey, C. C., et al. (1999). "Schizotypal Personality Disorder and MRI Abnormalities of Temporal Lobe Gray Matter." *Biological Psychiatry* 45: 1393–1402.

Farmer, C. M., et al. (2000). "Visual Perception and Working Memory in Schizotypal Personality." *American Journal of Psychiatry* 157: 781–786.

"Schizotypal Personality Physical Abnormalities Studied." (2000). *Brown University Child and Adolescent Behavior Letter* 16(4): 4.

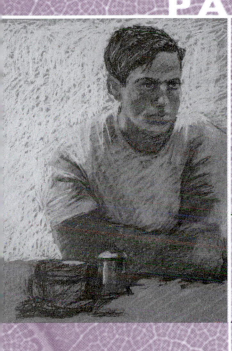

PART SIX

The Client Experiencing a Somatoform, Factitious, or Dissociative Disorder

Andre

EASY

GENDER

M

AGE

52

SETTING

- Outpatient surgery suite

ETHNICITY

- White American

CULTURAL CONSIDERATIONS

- French

PREEXISTING CONDITION

COEXISTING CONDITION

- Periodic chest and jaw pain

COMMUNICATION

DISABILITY

SOCIOECONOMIC

- Middle-class college professor

SPIRITUAL/RELIGIOUS

- Catholic

PHARMACOLOGIC

Omeprazole (Prilosec)

PSYCHOSOCIAL

- Has no known friends
- Has no close relatives
- Isolates self except for contacts with students, medical personnel, and periodic contact with priests

ETHICAL

- Reading the chart of a client not assigned to you: a client you are curious about because you know this client outside the health care setting

ALTERNATIVE THERAPY

PRIORITIZATION

DELEGATION

HYPOCHONDRIASIS

Level of difficulty: Easy

Overview: Requires critical thinking, patience, empathy, knowledge, and skill in therapeutic communication skills as well as acknowledging and addressing whether a dual relationship with a client is ethical or not.

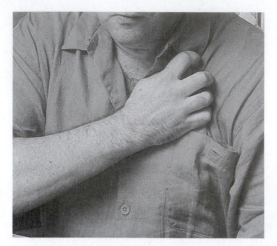

Client Profile

Andre is a 52-year-old college professor who was born in France. He came to the United States as a young man to attend college. After graduation, he returned to France for a number of years. Later, he decided to accept a teaching position at a small college in the United States. He teaches several chemistry classes designed for pre-med and nursing students. Some of the students ask a lot of questions, which causes him to think these particular students must be quite dense. While there could be other reasons for their inquisitiveness, those reasons escape him. Andre is sometimes overwhelmed by the amount of preparation and grading he must do.

Andre never married. Shortly after he came to the United States, his father died unexpectedly. He has no known friends or family that he is close to. Over the past several months, he has periodically experienced chest pain and sometimes notices he feels strange when he bends over. He is preoccupied with this chest pain and is becoming more impatient with his students. The students, who had already complained to the Dean about his manner before the chest pain began, are complaining even more. The students also complained that he is too serious and never smiles. The Dean advises Andre to be more sensitive to the students' needs. Andre asks himself, "How can I, when I am so sick?"

Andre finally sees his health care provider, who orders an electrocardiogram. It is evaluated as normal. Andre is not sufficiently reassured and continues to worry about the possibility of a heart attack. He then calls the clinic to tell the triage nurse that he is still experiencing some periodic chest pain and jaw pain. The triage nurse immediately schedules an appointment for that day with one of the health care providers. A stress ECG is done. Some slight irregularities justify a referral to a cardiac specialist. After reviewing the test results and a physical and history, the specialist suggests cardiac catheterization to determine the patency of the major cardiac vessels.

Case Study

Andre presents himself to the outpatient surgery suite for the surgical procedure. After receiving his preoperative medication, he recognizes a familiar voice calling his name. It is one of his nursing students from chemistry class: one of the ones who asks a lot of questions and smiles all the time. Andre does not smile back; she thinks he is too serious and even rude. The student nurse explains that she is in outpatient surgery for a one-day observational experience. After surgery, he looks around to see if the nursing student is still there. When he doesn't see her, he thinks perhaps he imagined she was there. The cardiac surgeon explains that the cardiac catheterization findings, saying, "You have 30 percent occlusion of one major heart vessel, but this is nothing to worry about."

In a follow-up visit, the cardiac surgeon suggests the chest pain might be due to heartburn, possibly gastroesophageal reflux disease (GERD). He recommends consulting his primary health care provider for evaluation, who might prescribe some omeprazole (Prilosec). Andre conveys his belief that he has a serious heart condition that is just not showing up. The surgeon begins to think about the possibility of Hypochondrias. Andre buys some over-the-counter omeprazole and takes it on his own.

Two days later, Andre calls the triage nurse saying, "I am still having chest pain. I really think I might have a serious cardiac problem that the health care providers are missing. Perhaps you could get me an appointment with another health care provider in the clinic?"

Questions

1. If you were the nursing student in this case and saw your current professor's name on the outpatient surgery list on a day you are assigned to observe in outpatient surgery, what would you do and why? What if you were a nurse working in outpatient surgery and Andre was your neighbor? Is Andre being rude when he does not smile back?

2. Is it all right for the student nurse to read her professor's chart? Should any nurse read an acquaintance's chart?

Questions (continued)

3. What should the triage nurse say or do when the professor asks for an appointment with another health care provider?

4. What are the criteria for a diagnosis of Hypochondriasis? Does this client meet these criteria?

5. A colleague asks you, "How is a client with Hypochondriasis different than a client with Somatization Disorder or Conversion Disorder?" What answer would you give?

6. What are the cause, incidence, and course of Hypochondriasis?

7. What are clients with Hypochondriasis like?

8. What treatment modalities are being used with clients who have Hypochondriasis?

9. What assessment data are needed for this client? What is the development task (according to Erickson) for this client's age and stage? Why is it important to assess where this client is in resolving this task?

10. What nursing diagnoses, goals, and interventions would you write for this client?

Questions and Suggested Answers

1. If you were the nursing student in this case and saw your current professor's name on the outpatient surgery list on a day you are assigned to observe in outpatient surgery, what would you do and why? What if you were a nurse working in outpatient surgery and Andre was your neighbor? Is Andre being rude when he does not smile back? As the student nurse, you need to immediately notify your instructor of your student–teacher relationship with this client, which, if combined with a nursing relationship, constitutes a dual relationship. Although there is nothing in most (or perhaps all) nursing practice acts about dual relationships, it is a matter of ethical concern. Some professional licensing boards prohibit those they license from having dual relationships. The student–professor relationship is one in which the professor has power over the student; now the power has changed, and there is a second relationship superimposed on the first. You should switch places with another student for the day or ask to be scheduled in areas away from the professor.

It is advisable for nurses not to care for neighbors, close friends, or relatives in hospitals or other professional settings in the role of a hospital employee or a student in clinical rotation at the hospital. The ability to be objective and therapeutic might be compromised by the first relationship. Avoiding involvement in dual relationships helps protect the nurse from accusations of breach of confidentiality and helps the client feel more secure that someone who knows him outside of the hospital setting won't breach confidentiality.

According to Lawless (2006), there is a common myth that the French people are rude. This myth seems to arise from the serious countenance of the French and their failure to smile back when others smile at them. Smiling only when it is meant is a French cultural practice. While Americans tend to smile frequently and at everyone, the French are more reserved. This difference in cultural practice is often mistaken for rudeness. The French cultural tendency to be reserved might contribute to the professor's isolation, especially when others do not understand why he does not smile at them.

2. Is it all right for the student nurse to read her professor's chart? Should any nurse read an acquaintance's chart? It is unethical for the student to read the professor's chart out of curiosity, even if she keeps what she learns confidential. Students are usually allowed to read hospital charts for educational purposes, but not to satisfy their curiosity about any client, regardless of whether or not they have a relationship of any kind with that client. It also is unethical for a nurse to read the chart of a neighbor or social acquaintance out of curiosity.

3. What should the triage nurse needs to say or do when the professor professor asks for an appointment with another health care provider? A number of acceptable answers exist for this question. This situation calls for critical thinking. Clients are able to fire their primary care provider and select another one. On the other hand, it is not helpful for someone who might have Hypochondriasis to shop until he finds someone who will do another invasive procedure or unnecessary treatment that could harm him.

The triage nurse, believing the client has Hypochondriasis, could say to the client, "I hear you saying you would like to change your health care provider. You can do this at anytime; however, your current provider is already familiar with your case. What about giving your provider one more chance to work with you? Then, you can tell your provider yourself that you are thinking of switching to someone else and why."

On the other hand, the triage nurse might consider the possibility that Andre has a medical problem that is being missed such as cancer of the esophageal gastric junction. It can cause pain in the area of the heart from reflux, and this pain can feel like a heart attack. GERD without cancer also can create pain that feels like a heart attack. Pain in the jaw can be from heart attack, or it can be from dental problems or even grinding the teeth at night while asleep. The side effects listed for Omeprazole (Spratto and Woods, 2006, 965), which the client is taking for heartburn, include angina, chest pain, tachycardia, bradycardia, and palpitation.

4. What are the criteria for a diagnosis of Hypochondriasis? Does this client meet these criteria?

Criteria for Hypochondriasis	Does Client Meet the Criteria?
Based on a faulty interpretation of body symptoms, the person is preoccupied with the fear of having or already having a serious disease.	Yes, the client fears he has a serious heart condition that his health care providers have missed.
Even with appropriate medical evaluation and reassurance, the client's preoccupation with having a serious disease, or getting one, persists.	Yes, the client has had an electrocardiogram, stress test, and cardiac catheterization yet still believes he has a serious heart condition that is being missed.
There is not delusional intensity to faulty interpretation of body symptoms or preoccupation about disease or only a concern about appearance.	Yes, the professor can admit the possibility that there might be no disease at all, but he remains preoccupied.
Preoccupation causes clinically significant distress in important area(s) of functioning such as social, educational, occupational, or other.	Yes, the professor has become impatient with students; the Dean has told the professor to improve.
Disturbance duration is at least six months.	Probably, our case says "for several months." Clarification is needed.
The preoccupation cannot be explained better by General Anxiety Disorder, Obsessive-Compulsive Disorder, Panic Disorder, Major Depressive Episode, Separation Anxiety, or another Somatoform Disorder.	This area needs assessment.

Adapted from the *Diagnostic and Statistical Manual of Mental Disorders* (APA, 2000).

5. A colleague asks you, "How is a client with Hypochondriasis different than a client with Somatization Disorder or Conversion Disorder?" What answer would you give? In Hypochondriasis, the person misinterprets body symptoms, building them up into a serious disease, or fears he has a serious disease. A client with Somatization Disorder has a history of many physical complaints involving at least four pain symptoms, two gastrointestinal symptoms, one sexual symptom, and one pseudo-neurologic symptom before age 30. A client with Conversion Disorder unconsciously deals with a conflict by having a physical symptom with no medical explanation for the symptom. In this case, Andre might actually have GERD or heartburn that accounts for his chest pain, which he has magnified into a serious heart condition. It is always important to keep an open mind, as the client could be correct that he has a serious disease that is being missed.

6. What are the cause, incidence, and course of Hypochondriasis? While the cause of Hypochondriasis (HC) is unknown, Hilty and associates (2005) suggest the possibility of developmental and other predisposing factors such as parental attitudes about disease, previous experience with physical disease, and culturally acquired attitudes as contributing factors. The cognitive model of HC views the client as amplifying somatic sensations and having a lower threshold for discomfort than most others. Social learning theory looks at the possibility that the client with HC is subconsciously welcoming a sick role to avoid unpleasant obligations and duties. A neurochemical model looks at the similarities and overlaps between HC and other Somatoform Disorders and depressive and anxiety disorders and suggests a possible biologic cause or factor. Noyes and associates (2005, 110) studied 602 veterans who had served in the Gulf War and found "negative temperament or neuroticism is strongly associated with hypochondriacal concerns." They further state that "Hypochondriasis appears to be within the domain of personality. . . . It remains for future research to show whether negative temperament is a vulnerability factor for hypochondriasis or hypochondiasis is itself a personality disorder."

The prevalence of HC is estimated at 1–5 percent in the general population and 2–7 percent in primary care outpatients (APA, 2000). Hilty and associates (2005) describe the frequency of HC at 0.08–4.5 percent in primary care settings. They state that a third of the clients with HC will eventually experience significant improvement. Hypochondriasis is often episodic, with some quiescent periods and equally long periods of Hypochondriasis. The disorder can last month to years. Hypochondriasis can begin at any age with onset typically believed to occur in early adulthood (APA, 2000).

7. What are clients with Hypochondriasis like? In addition to fearing having a serious disease based on misinterpretation of bodily signs and sensations, clients excessively seek medical tests to verify having a serious illness as well as treatment for serious illness. Health care provider shopping and frustration and anger on the part of both client and provider are common, as no serious illness is typically discovered (APA, 2000). On the other hand, Abramowitz and colleagues (2002) describe a subset of clients with Hypochondriasis who believe they are seriously ill and avoid seeing medical personnel fearing they will receive an upsetting evaluation. Noyes and associates (2002, 503) state, "Fear of death appears to be an integral part of Hypochondriasis." This finding carries implications for the nurse, suggesting a need to assess the client in regard to fear of death as well as fear of separation and purpose in life.

Frisch and Frisch (2006, 443–444) point out that some clients with Hypochondriasis "focus their concerns on a single disease (cancer or heart disease) and seek confirmation of their fears in minimal symptoms or alterations of normal bodily function," while others are focused on a variety of symptoms (e.g., a cough or a missed heart beat). Reassurance after examination and tests does not help or only helps temporarily. Frisch and Frisch conclude that worries about health "tend to become a major focus of the individual's life and daily routine "Frisch and Frisch (2006, 443–444).

Edward Walker at the University of Washington studied people with Hypochondriasis and concluded his subjects usually felt a lack of control over illness, were unmarried, and possibly looked for social support from health care providers although they were often wary of health care providers for good reasons such as being abused as children (Polera, 1998).

8. What treatment modalities are being used with clients who have Hypochondriasis? Hilty and colleagues (2005) report that clients diagnosed with Hypochondriasis seem to have a greater chance of improvement if they have high socioeconomic status, receive treatment for any anxiety and/or depression present, and do not have a personality disorder. They describe treatment for Hypochondriasis as consisting of psychotherapy plus antidepressants when depression is present. Walker suggests that a psychiatric evaluation and compassion from health care providers are needed (Polera, 1998). The literature (Abramowitz et al., 2002) often recommends Cognitive Behavioral Therapy.

Treatment includes supportive care, such as staying in regular contact with provider, medication such as antidepressants and antianxiety drugs, and psychotherapy to change thinking and behavior (Cleveland Clinic, 2005).

9. What assessment data are needed for this client? What is the development task (according to Erickson) for this client's age and stage? Why is it important to assess where this client is in resolving this task? The nurse developing a care plan will want to gather a physical and mental health history. It is important to list all medications that this client is taking and how much he is taking. He could be overusing the omaprazole. The nurse must review the side effects of this medication to see if they relate to any of Andre's complaints. The nurse also will want to gather information about Andre's relationship with his father and the effect of his death. A mood assessment is indicated to determine if any depression or anxiety is present. The nurse needs to gather data on this client's social contacts (and potential social contacts) as well as the client's spiritual needs and relationships with the Church.

At age 52, Andre is in the ego integrity versus despair stage of development according to Erickson. This is a time of internal struggle and life review in which a person age 45 and older looks at his life and decides if he has been successful or if he could have done things better, differently, or more. If Andre has fallen into despair about his life accomplishments not measuring up, he might hold contempt for himself. He needs to be assessed for where he is in resolving his developmental task, as this has implications for goals and interventions. If Andre is resolving this task or has resolved it, then positive reinforcement will be helpful. If he is in despair, then he needs help reframing (taking a different look) at his life and accomplishments and gaining a greater sense of comfort in what he has accomplished.

10. What nursing diagnoses, goals, and interventions would you write for this client? Nursing goals will generally focus on changing thinking and behavior. Goals could address spending less time in seeking medical help and being in the ill role and more time on doing other things. Another goal might be for the client to state feeling increased understanding and control over signs and symptoms. It would be appropriate to include goals related to increasing diversional activities and social contacts.

Nursing diagnoses could include Powerless over illness and death and other areas of life; Fear of illness and/or dying; Social isolation; Chronic low self-esteem; Ineffective coping; Knowledge deficit; and Deficient diversional activity.

Possible interventions could include

- Develop a trusting supportive/adversarial relationship with client.
- Mirror the client's serious expression, as this will likely feel more comfortable to the client.
- Teach the client about symptoms, and encourage the client to research symptoms to include possible normal physiologic reasons as well as serious problems.
- Include Cognitive Behavioral Therapy in treatment, and work with the therapist and client; teach/reinforce avoidance of thinking errors such as magnifying signs and symptoms and catastrophizing.
- Listen respectfully to client.
- Encourage client to talk about accomplishments and goals and see value in his work.
- Encourage the client to talk about his fears, including fear of death. Encourage client to talk with his priest about his purpose in life and any fears related to death and dying.
- Seek input from the client about ideas for dealing with fears (this promotes commitment to following through and decreases feelings of powerlessness).

References

Abramowitz, J. S., et al. (2002). "A Contemporary Conceptual Model of Hypochondriasis." *Mayo Clinic Proceedings* 77(12): 1323–1330.

American Psychiatric Association (APA). (2000). *Diagnostic and Statistical Manual of Mental Disorders, 4th ed.* Text Revision. Washington, DC: American Psychiatric Association.

Cleveland Clinic. (2005). "Hypochondriasis." www.clevelandclinic.org/health/health-info/docs/3700/3783.asp?index=9886. Accessed February 2, 2005.

Frisch, N. C. and L. E. Frisch. (2006). *Psychiatric Mental Health Nursing, 3d ed.* Albany, NY: Thomson Delmar Learning.

Hilty, D. M., et al. (2005). "Hypochondriasis." www.emedicine.com/MED/topic3122.htm. Accessed June 13, 2006.

——. Hypochondriasis. www.clevelandclinic.org/health/health-info/docs/3700/3783.asp?index=9886. Accessed February 2, 2005.

Lawless, L. K. (2006). "The Rude French Myth." http://french.about.com/cs/culture/a/rudefrench.htm. Accessed February 7, 2006.

Noyes, R., Jr., et al. (2002). "Hypochondriasis and Fear of Death." *Journal of Nervous and Mental Disease* 190(8): 503–509.

Noyes, R., Jr., et al. (2005). "Relationship Between Hypochondriacal Concerns and Personality Dimensions and Traits in a Military Population." *Journal of Nervous and Mental Disease* 193(2): 110–118.

Polera, C. (1998). "Help for Hypochondriacs: How Physicians Deal with Patients Who Are Psychologically Dependent on Them." *Psychology Today* 31(2): 14.

Spratto, G. R. and A. L. Woods. (2006). *PDR Nurse's Drug Handbook.* Clifton Park, NJ: Thomson Delmar Learning.

CASE STUDY 2

Alyssa

GENDER

F

AGE

24

SETTING

- Office of a plastic surgeon

ETHNICITY

- White American

CULTURAL CONSIDERATIONS

PREEXISTING CONDITION

COEXISTING CONDITION

COMMUNICATION

DISABILITY

SOCIOECONOMIC

- Lives with upper-class parents

SPIRITUAL/RELIGIOUS

PHARMACOLOGIC

PSYCHOSOCIAL

- Focuses on perceived body flaws and desire for plastic surgery, not on interpersonal relationships

LEGAL

- Need for a female staff member present in examination room when a male health care provider examines a disrobed female

ETHICAL

- If demand for plastic surgery is driven by a psychiatric condition, is it ethical to help prepare the client for plastic surgery?

ALTERNATIVE THERAPY

PRIORITIZATION

DELEGATION

MODERATE

SOMATOFORM, FACTITIOUS, OR DISSOCIATIVE DISORDERS

Level of difficulty: Moderate

Overview: Requires knowledge, interpersonal skills, empathy, understanding, critical thinking, and therapeutic communication skills. The nurse must motivate the client to get professional psychiatric assessment and therapy prior to further discussions with the surgeon about another plastic surgery.

Client Profile

Alyssa is a 24-year-old female who was raised in an upper-class, two-parent family. She was a high school cheerleader who often obsessed over a pimple on her face or an imagined wrinkle. After high-school graduation, she married the guy voted best looking in her class. Two years later, her husband divorced her for "someone better looking." Since that time, Alyssa has been looking into reflective surfaces more and becoming increasingly concerned about parts of her body. She now dislikes the shape of her buttocks. She thinks they look too flat, calling herself "Ms. No Butt." While projecting a joking attitude about her perceived lack of gluteal muscle, Alyssa actually is very concerned about her "ugly butt." She decides to see a plastic surgeon to have some fat injected into her buttocks. Friends and family members tell her that she does not need this work, but she is convinced that she does.

This is not Alyssa's first plastic surgery. While friends and family members spend money on entertainment and vacations, Alyssa spends her money on cosmetic surgery. She even has credit card debt attributable to her nose job, chin implant, brow lift, and breast enlargement. She has been so busy studying her body flaws and trying to fix them that she cannot hold down a job; she must live with her parents.

Alyssa plans to get the money for this surgery from her parents by requesting it as a "birthday present for the next ten years." If the birthday approach does not work, she will ask them for a loan.

Case Study

Alyssa makes an appointment with a plastic surgeon. After taking a history, the plastic surgeon tells the client he will need to take some body measurements and photographs. The nurse instructs her about what clothing to remove and assures her that she (the nurse) will be in the room when the plastic surgeon does the measurements. The client says, "No, I don't need you there. You have other work to do." After the measurements and photographs, the plastic surgeon tells Alyssa that before any plastic surgery can be done, she needs to get a thorough physical examination by her primary caretaker, make an appointment with a licensed mental health professional for counseling at least once a week for ten weeks, and get an assessment by a psychiatrist. The plastic surgeon does not verbally deny her the surgery or tell her it is an outrageous idea, but simply requests she complete this preliminary preparation first and then discusses a possible surgery date twelve weeks from this visit. When the health care provider leaves the examining room, Alyssa looks at herself in the mirror and then in the reflection of a stainless steel cabinet. She turns to the nurse and asks, "Does the surgeon think I am crazy? Is he going to do this surgery or not?"

Questions

1. If you were the nurse in the plastic surgeon's office, how would you respond when Alyssa says you do not need to be present in the examination room? How would you respond to her last question?

2. Why do you think the plastic surgeon made the recommendations he did? Are clients with Body Dysmorphic Disorder (BDD) generally satisfied with their cosmetic surgery?

3. What is BDD? Does this client meet the diagnostic criteria for BDD?

4. What causes BDD?

5. What is the prevalence of BDD? Do many males get this disorder? If so, are there gender-based differences in the body parts seen as flawed?

6. What is the usual course of BDD? Are any comorbid conditions common?

7. What effect, if any, did this client's culture have on development of BDD?

8. Do all nurses need to know about BDD? If so, why?

9. What behaviors does the client with BDD exhibit?

10. What are the current treatments for BDD?

11. What questions should the nurse ask in gathering data on clients who have signs or symptoms of BDD?

12. What nursing diagnoses would you write for this client? What additional diagnoses might you encounter in clients with BDD? What interventions would you initiate?

Questions and Suggested Answers

1. If you were the nurse in the plastic surgeon's office, how would you respond when Alyssa says you do not need to be present in the examination room? How would you respond to her last question? You need to be present when the surgeon is with the client in order to protect the health care provider from any untrue accusations. You also need to be present to protect the client from any unprofessional behavior on the part of the health care provider. You must hold firm on the necessity of you being present when the health care provider examines the client. You might say, "It's an office rule that the nurse must be present during the examination." Or, you could say, "I have to help the health care provider with a few things during the examination." For his own legal protection, a male health care provider should never examine a female client without a female staff present.

You must answer the client's question about whether or not the health care provider thinks she is crazy and will do the surgery therapeutically. You could ask, "How much do you want this surgery?" When the client responds, you could add, "Do you want it badly enough to see your primary health care provider, a psychiatrist, and a therapist?" You also could ask, "What worries you the most about seeing your health care provider, a psychiatrist, and a therapist?" The idea is to gain insight about the client's concerns and establish trust. The client might be reluctant to see a psychiatrist or resistant to therapy for fear she will be diagnosed with a mental problem or that these professionals will see her as ugly. This client also might view anything other than cosmetic surgery as unnecessary. You need to support the plastic surgeon's request for preliminary assessment and therapy prior to plastic surgery.

If the client has Body Dysmorphic Disorder (BDD), plastic surgery will not improve her self-esteem or confidence. The client will likely be dissatisfied with the surgery results. The client's reaction to the plastic surgeon's request could range from mild concern to extreme anger. The nurse's response must be carefully calculated, with the tone and volume nonjudgmental, nonthreatening, calm, and soothing. If not, the client might opt to find another plastic surgeon who will do the surgery without psychiatric assessment or therapy.

2. Why do you think the plastic surgeon made the recommendations he did? Are clients with BDD generally satisfied with their cosmetic surgery?
Ethically, the plastic surgeon should not operate on a client with BDD. Such clients are often dissatisfied when the surgery is complete. They typically return and insist on corrections to the surgery. They often are angry that the surgery did not achieve what they imagined it would. The plastic surgeon is right to require reassurance that Alyssa is competent to make this decision and has sound reasons for doing so from both an ethical and legal standpoint.

Therapy can help Alyssa improve her self-esteem and body image and improve her problem-solving and financial management skills. The psychiatrist can determine if the client is mentally prepared to make a sound decision and benefit from cosmetic surgery or if this decision will only exacerbate her mental and physical condition. If the client has BDD, she will benefit more from psychological help than cosmetic surgery.

Getting the client to accept help will challenge the nurse's abilities. According to Renshaw (2003), people with BDD rarely see a psychiatrist or mental health professional and are offended if referred. Ashraf (2000, 2055) found that over half the subjects with BDD became preoccupied with another body part after surgery, adding "[e]ven if surgery resolved a BDD problem, patients were still 'significantly handicapped' by new-found complaints."

3. What is BDD? Does this client meet the diagnostic criteria for BDD?
In BDD, a person is preoccupied with a defect in her appearance. This defect can be a real anomaly blown out of proportion or imagined. The person experiences significant distress or impairment in important areas of functioning such as social or occupational. BDD must not be due to another mental disorder such as Anorexia Nervosa. BDD was once known

as dysmorphophobia, a term introduced in the late 1800s to described a condition in which a person has a pathologic concern for appearance (Anderson and Black, 2003).

Alyssa's signs and symptoms appear to match all the criteria for this disorder based on the comparison presented in the table below. In order to be diagnosed as having Body Dysmorphic Disorder, the client must meet all three criteria.

Criteria for Diagnosis of BDDr	Client's Signs/Symptoms
Preoccupation with a defect in appearance that is imagined or represents overconcern for a slight physical anomaly.	Yes, the client is preoccupied with appearance. She looks into reflective surfaces frequently and now seeks plastic surgery for a "flat derriere." She has undergone plastic surgery for things she sees as defects but others see as normal or near normal.
Preoccupation with a real or imagined defect causes great distress or impairment in one or more areas of life including, but not limited to, social, occupational, educational, or relational.	Yes, the client is experiencing distress in financial and interpersonal areas.
Preoccupation is not caused by another mental disorder such as Anorexia Nervosa, where the client is dissatisfied with body shape and size.	This must be determined via therapy and psychological testing.

Adapted from the *Diagnostic and Statistical Manual of Mental Disorders* (APA, 2000).

4. What causes BDD? Most theories suggest that BDD is a multifactorial, complex disorder involving both biologic and environmental factors. Anderson and Black (2003) state that a dysfunctional background and unfavorable childhood experiences such as teasing might cause the low self-esteem and insecurity that predispose a person to BDD. A case also could be made for a biologic predisposition, with environmental factors and low self-esteem triggering the biologic events that cause BDD.

Some recent theories suggest that BDD is associated with pathology of the frontal lobes of the brain, similar to pathology seen in clients with Obsessive Compulsive Disorder. In addition, a serotonergic dysfunction also is proposed (St. John, 2003).

5. What is the prevalence of BDD? Do many males get this disorder? If so, are there gender-based differences in the body parts seen as flawed? BDD affects about 2 percent of Americans and 6–15 percent of dermatology and cosmetic surgery patients: men and women equally and half [of the people with this disorder] have consulted a dermatologist or cosmetic surgeon and many have undergone at least one plastic surgery (St. John, 2003). Castle and colleagues (2004) report rates of BDD in persons seeking plastic surgery as falling between 7 percent and 15 percent.

Clients with BDD come from all economic and social strata in society. There are no "typical" demographics (Olivardia, 2002; Phillips, 2000).

Women seem preoccupied with the size and shape of breasts, hips, and legs as well as their body weight. Men focus on the size of their genitals, their height, amount of body hair, body build, and thinning scalp hair (Anderson and Black, 2003; St. John, 2003).

St. John (2003) purports that men are more likely than women to have muscle dysmorphia, also called "bigorexia" or "reverse anorexia." It involves a preoccupation with a distorted image of body size and muscle development. Whether clients with muscle dysmorphia have BDD or a form of BDD is unclear; however, St. John points out that these clients spend at least three hours a day in thoughts about their muscularity and avoid social activities while seeming to have little or no control over excessive weightlifting, attention to dietary regimens, and steroid abuse.

Renshaw (2003) relates that men are mainly preoccupied with the idea that their penis is too small. Interestingly, Renshaw suggests education can help prevent this condition, pointing out that a small penis in erection increases four times in size while a large penis will increase only two times in size. According to Renshaw, men or women seeking a sex change have total body dysmorphia.

6. What is the usual course of BDD? Are any comorbid conditions common? BDD usually starts in adolescence; however, it can present in childhood. Often, the person with BDD hides the symptoms and can go years without being diagnosed; some people are never diagnosed. The course is fairly continuous, with few or no periods without symptoms. The symptoms can be more or less intense at times. The body part of concern might change from time to time.

Clients with BDD commonly have other comorbid disorders including social phobia, Obsessive Compulsive Disorder (constant looking in the mirror or skin picking are the compulsions), and Major Depression. Olivardia (2002) states that 80 percent of the clients with BDD have underlying depression; mood and anxiety disorders including OCD also are common. A family history of BDD is not uncommon. St. John (2003) and Phillips (2000) both claim that 50 percent or more of the clients with BDD can also meet the criteria for Delusional Disorder, Somatic Type and might have ideas of reference that seem psychotic. Some clients also exhibit odd behaviors and social avoidance.

7. What effect, if any, did this client's culture have on development of BDD?
White Americans focus on appearance. A person's worth is often measured in how good-looking or young-looking he or she is. Americans are becoming increasingly dissatisfied with some part of their physical appearance as evidenced by the finding that in the United States, cosmetic procedures have increased by 66 percent since 1998 and 119 percent since 1997 (Castle et al., 2004).

In this culture, especially among persons in the upper middle class and above, plastic surgery is not only readily available but also seen as desirable. Moreover, divorce is common in this culture; in this client's case, divorce reinforced her idea that she was not attractive.

8. Do all nurses need to know about BDD? If so, why? All nurses, regardless of where they practice, need to know about BDD. Clients with BDD can be encountered in any setting, although they tend to seek out dermatologists and plastic surgeons and avoid mental health practitioners.

9. What behaviors does the client with BDD exhibit? Clients with BDD tend to look into any reflective surface (mirror, puddle, glass surface, appliance surface, etc.) or go out of their way to avoid seeing their reflection. They seek almost constant reassurance about their appearance and others' perceptions of their flaws. Clients might measure body parts frequently, compare themselves to others, engage in skin picking, groom excessively, camouflage perceived defects, and change clothing frequently. These clients tend to seek unnecessary dermatologic and plastic surgery procedures (Phillips, 2000).

Clients with BDD are perfectionists, exhibit low self-esteem, and an estimated 80 percent have symptoms of depression (Olivardia, 2002). Clients with perfectionism might become anxious if things are not ordered well or spend inordinate amounts of time getting their clothing to look just right. A person with underlying depression might manifest a negative attitude or a flattened affect.

10. What are the current treatments for BDD? Ashraf (2000, 2055), quoting a child and adolescent psychiatrist, states, "Treatments [for BDD] currently include selective serotonin reuptake inhibitors (SSRIs), augmentation with low-dose neuroleptics, and cognitive and behavioural therapy."

Phillips (2000) identifies SSRI therapy as the first-line approach for severe cases, recommending that Cognitive Behavioral Therapy be used in combination with the psychopharmacology. He calls for intensive, frequent sessions with periodic maintenance sessions. Phillips points out that one SSRI might be more effective than another, suggesting a medication change if a particular SSRI is not effective. He advises that pharmacotherapy should continue for twelve to sixteen weeks; if effective, it should continue at least one year. For mild cases of BDD without significant comorbidity, Phillips recommends Cognitive Behavioral Therapy as the first-line approach.

11. What questions should the nurse ask in gathering data on clients who have signs or symptoms of BDD? The nurse should ask the following questions:

- What plastic surgeons have done surgery on you in the past? What are the types and dates of each surgery? (Helps determine client's degree of preoccupation with dissatisfaction with body parts. Highlights client's tendency to change health care providers frequently.)
- On a scale of 1 to10, how satisfied were you with the results of each surgery? (Clients with BDD are usually not satisfied with results of surgeries.)
- What are your expectations for any future surgeries? (Indicates whether or not expectations are reasonable.)
- What crises do you have in your life now? (Clients with BDD tend to have crises.)
- What do you say to yourself when you look into the mirror? (Helps establish whether or not client avoids mirrors and has a distorted body image.)

In addition, Phillips (2000) suggests asking five additional questions: "(1) Are you very worried about your appearance in any way? If yes, what are your concerns? (2) Do any concerns about your appearance preoccupy you thoughts? If you add up all the time you worry about your appearance in a day, how much time would that be? (3) What effect, if any, does your periodic preoccupation with appearances have on your life? (4) Has your appearance brought you distress or affected areas of your life and/or (5) affected relationships with family or friends?"

12. What nursing diagnoses would you write for this client? What additional diagnoses might you encounter in clients with BDD? What interventions would you initiate? The nursing diagnoses could include:

- Body image disturbed
- Chronic low self-esteem
- Anxiety
- Social interaction impaired

Some clients might have findings that warrant a diagnosis of Risk for self-directed violence. As many as 25–30 percent of clients with BDD attempt suicide; they also are at risk for auto accidents due to inattention to their driving and injuries from surgeries they perform on themselves to correct perceived flaws (St. Johns, 2003, 18).

As an office nurse for a plastic surgeon, your contact with this client would be limited. Opportunities for additional contact could occur if you convey a caring attitude and ask her to call back and let you know what she has decided about the surgeon's recommendations. You can encourage her to get therapy and give verbal reinforcement if she does. In subsequent calls or office visits, you can encourage her to take any SSRI or other medication ordered for her. You could instruct the client in thought-stopping and relaxation techniques. Education on problem-solving process and modeling problem solving would help the client reduce crises.

When the client talks about dissatisfaction with a prior surgery, you could change the subject or distract the client rather than reinforcing this idea. You can encourage the client to learn leisure activities skills. While trained professionals should do therapy, the office nurse can become knowledgeable about the approaches used and support these interventions.

References

American Psychiatric Association (APA). (2000). *Diagnostic and Statistical Manual of Mental Disorders, 4th ed.* Text Revision. Washington, DC: American Psychiatric Association.

Anderson, R. C. and J. Black. (2003). "Body Dysmorphic Disorder: Recognition and Treatment." *Plastic Surgical Nursing* 23(3): 125–131.

Ashraf, L. (2000). "Surgery Offers Little Help for Patients with Body Dysmorphic Disorder." *Lancet* 355(9220): 2055.

Castle, D. J., et al. (2004), "Correlates of Dysmorphic Concern in People Seeking Cosmetic Enhancement." *Australian New Zealand Journal of Psychiatry* 36(6): 436–444.

Olivardia, R. (2002). "Body Image Obsession in Men." *Healthy Weight Journal* 16(4): 59–64.

Phillips, K. A. (2000). "Body Dysmorphic Disorder: Diagnostic Controversies and Treatment Challenges." *Bulletin of Menninger Clinic* 64(1): 18–35.

Renshaw, D. C. (2003). "Body Dysmorphia, the Plastic Surgeon and the Psychiatrist." *Psychiatric Times* 20(7): 64–66.

St. John, D. (2003). "Imagined Ugliness: Body Dysmorphic Disorder." *Physician Assistant* 27(7): 15–26.

CASE STUDY 3

Wanda

GENDER

F

AGE

28

SETTING

- General medical hospital inpatient unit

ETHNICITY

- White American

CULTURAL CONSIDERATIONS

- French Canadian

PREEXISTING CONDITION

COEXISTING CONDITION

COMMUNICATION

DISABILITY

SOCIOECONOMIC

SPIRITUAL/RELIGIOUS

PHARMACOLOGIC

- Meperidine (Demerol)
- Ibuprofen (Motrin)
- Lorazepam (Ativan)
- Naloxone (Narcan)

PSYCHOSOCIAL

- Separated from husband and son

LEGAL

- Client's right to medication ordered

ETHICAL

- Obligation to do no harm requires assessment before giving pain medication

ALTERNATIVE THERAPY

- Meditation
- Exercise

PRIORITIZATION

DELEGATION

- Medication administration
- Bath and hygiene care

DIFFICULT

PAIN DISORDER

Level of difficulty: High

Overview: Requires knowledge of Pain Disorder and critical thinking. The nurse must determine what assessments are needed; what findings are necessary for dispensing or withholding pain medication; and what client care tasks can be delegated to vocational/practical nurses and nursing assistants.

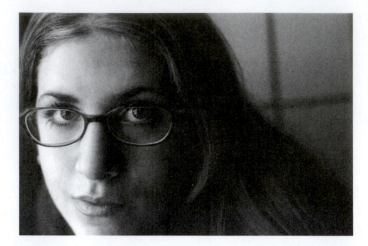

Client Profile

Wanda is a 28-year-old French Canadian female who came to the United States to visit her sister and ended up marrying, going to massage therapy school, and working as a massage therapist in a hotel spa. Life was difficult. Her marriage had a significant amount of fighting and making up. She disliked speaking English to customers, preferring her native French. After Wanda started having severe headaches and calling in sick, she lost her job. She began spending her days on the sofa and barely attended to the most basic needs of her 5-year-old son. Wanda and her husband separated. He claimed her entire focus was pain, saying that her constant visits to health care providers and emergency departments made it impossible for them to be together without pain or financial difficulties coming between them. He took their 5-year-old son and moved back with his parents, telling his sister-in-law that he doubted Wanda would even notice that they had left.

Case Study

Wanda's health care provider is admitting her to the medical unit of a medical-surgical hospital. Her chief complaint is severe headaches. Wanda tells the admitting nurse, "I am a massage therapist, but I haven't been able to work because of horrible headaches. I've tried sumatriptan (Imitrex), ergotamine (Ergostat), and dihydromergotamine (Migranal) nasal spray and nothing helps. Recently, I've been trying meditation and weekly massages."

The health care provider's history and physical notes indicate no brain pathology has been found to date, and the health care provider is considering a diagnosis of Pain Disorder. The health care provider orders meperidine (Demerol) 125 mg every three to four hours as needed for pain, ibuprofen (Motrin) 400 mg every four to six hours as needed for pain, lorazepam (Ativan) 1–2 mg as needed for agitation or insomnia (not to exceed 8 mg per day), a daily multiple vitamin, and daily birth control pill.

The next morning, the primary nurse enters Wanda's room at 7:30 AM to do an assessment. Wanda appears to be sleeping soundly. The nurse has difficulty awakening Wanda and manages to wake her just enough to get some vital signs. The vital signs are:

- Temperature: 97.6° F
- Respirations: 12
- Pulse: 68
- Blood pressure: 118/74 mm Hg

Wanda does not awaken for breakfast and appears to be asleep at 9 AM when the nurse tries again to arouse her for assessment, routine medications, and breakfast. The nurse calls her name several times and shakes the client. Wanda finally arouses and immediately says, "Nurse, I need my pain medication. My headache is very bad."

Questions

1. If you were Wanda's nurse, what would you think when Wanda is difficult to arouse and immediately asks for pain medication?

2. What must the nurse assess before making a decision about whether or not to give pain medication? Why are these assessments necessary?

3. Does the nurse need to wait until the pain level is high before giving medication? Why or why not? What else should the nurse assess in the assessment phase of the nursing process?

4. Would it be all right for Wanda's assigned nurse to delegate the administration of pain medication to another nurse? Can the bath and hygiene care be delegated? What factors should the nurse take into consideration when delegating aspects of Wanda's care?

5. What criteria must be met for a diagnosis of Pain Disorder? Do this client's behaviors match the criteria?

6. How would you start to build a therapeutic relationship with Wanda?

7. What psychological stressors and cultural influences might have contributed to Wanda's chronic pain?

8. What nursing diagnoses would you write for this client? What would be some likely short-term goals for this client?

9. What nursing interventions would be helpful?

10. What are the current treatments for chronic Pain Disorder?

Questions and Suggested Answers

1. If you were Wanda's nurse, what would you think when you have difficulty waking Wanda and she immediately asks for pain medication? A common reaction when a client asks for pain medication on awakening is suspicion that the client does not have pain. Another common reaction is anger toward the client for wanting medication she does not appear to need when the nurse is busy with other clients who have "real needs." You might be suspicious or angry; on the other hand, you might feel sorry for this client and her ongoing suffering and want to immediately give her more medication. You also could think this client is or will become addicted to pain medication. Many thoughts could cross you mind, based on your experiences with pain or those of family members, friends, or other clients. Other thoughts could arise out of your culture's view of pain (e.g., Northern European cultures tend to be stoic, while Americans tend to want a pill for every health problem).

You need to base your decision about what pain medication to give and when on assessment, not on your emotional reaction. Your voice tone, body language, and verbal response need to convey that you respect the client, are there to help her, and can be trusted to act in the client's best interests. If after your assessment you still question whether or not to give the pain medication, you should review your findings with your supervisor to make a decision. Ultimately, you are responsible for acting in a professional manner, using good judgment, and acting as a reasonable and prudent nurse would act. Frisch and Frisch (2006, 514) stress that nurses and treatment teams working with clients who have Pain Disorder must not become part of the problem by being "taken up in angry self-defeating relationships" with the client.

2. What must the nurse assess before making a decision about whether or not to give pain medication? Why are these assessments necessary? The nurse must assess location, type, duration, and level of pain before giving pain medication. The client usually needs to have some pain, although not necessarily a high level of pain, to justify giving the medication. This assessment also serves as a baseline for comparing the client's pain before and after medication administration as well as providing an ongoing picture of the client's pain level. Common tools for pain assessment include the Visual Analog Scale, the Number Intensity Scale, and the Descriptive Pain Intensity Scale. The Visual Analog Scale is a 10-cm line with "no pain" marked at one end and the "worst pain imaginable" at the other. Clients mark their pain severity along the scale where they think it would best fit. The Number Intensity Scale involves asking clients to rate their pain on a scale of 0 to 10 with 0 being no pain and 10 being the worst pain. The

Descriptive Scale asks clients to rate pain as mild, moderate, severe, very severe, or worst possible. King (2000) suggests no one scale seems better than the others. In addition, there are more comprehensive pain survey tools such as the McGill Pain Questionnaire, SF-36 Health Survey, and the Multiaxial Assessment of Pain.

In addition to pain assessment, the nurse must assess vital signs to ensure the client does not have respiratory depression. You will recall that the client had respirations of twelve the morning after admission. If this is still the case, the nurse must withhold any pain medication that would further depress respiration; the nurse must notify the charge nurse and the health care provider as well. The nurse needs to be aware that the health care provider might order naloxone (Narcan) to reverse the effects of any pain medication that depressed respirations. The nurse must be familiar with naloxone and know how to obtain it quickly.

If vital signs, including respirations, are within normal range, the nurse needs to review the order for pain medication and calculate how much pain medication the client has received in the past twenty-four hours, noting how long it has been since the client's last dose. The meperidine order specifies every three to four hours, and the nurse cannot give it sooner. Because meperidine can depress respiratory centers, dosing must not exceed the ordered amount. Prescribed amounts of ibuprofen taken should not exceed 50 mg/kg/day (Spratto and Woods, 2005).

The nurse should not delay meperidine when the client has an order for it, her respiratory status and other assessment findings are satisfactory, and the client has not reached the limits of safe dosing over the past twenty-four hours.

The client's level of anxiety must be assessed and considered along with all the information gathered about pain. She might need lorazepam instead, or in addition to, pain medication. Lorazepam is an antianxiety benzodiazepine and a controlled substance that reduces anxiety, decreases tension, and relaxes muscles, which could help reduce the headache pain. The question that must be answered is, "Does the client need anxiety relieved or pain relieved?" Further, the nurse is challenged to find ways to teach the client to relax and reduce anxiety by alternative means (e.g., music and relaxation therapy).

3. Does the nurse need to wait until the pain level is high before giving medication? Why or why not? What else should the nurse assess in the assessment phase of the nursing process? The client has a legal right to ordered pain medication as long as there is not a clear indication to withhold it. Yezierski and colleagues (2004) point out the importance of early recognition and treatment of a client's acute pain, saying that this reduces the chance that the central nervous system will become sensitized and develop chronic pain. They also suggest that once a client has chronic pain, even harmless stimuli can cause feelings of pain. This client already has chronic pain; however, the nurse should work on symptom management while assisting in discovering underlying causes and alternative or complementary approaches to dealing with this pain.

The nurse needs to assess all body systems, strengths, limitations, support systems, interests, talents, and spiritual and psychological strengths and needs. The more the nurse knows about the client, the clearer the nursing problems will be. Resolving some of the nursing problems might reduce the need for medication or help identify some means for reducing pain other than medication.

4. Would it be all right for Wanda's assigned nurse to delegate the administration of pain medication to another nurse? Can the bath and hygiene care be delegated? What factors should the nurse take into consideration when delegating aspects of Wanda's care? In the course of Wanda's care, there will be times when the primary nurse will need to delegate pain medication administration to another nurse; however, if at all possible, the primary nurse should personally assess the client's pain and administer the pain medication. This provides an opportunity for the nurse to build a relationship with the client, assess what is going on with her, and suggest new ways of thinking about and dealing with the pain.

Every interaction with this client is an important opportunity to do assessment and build trust. You might delegate the personal hygiene assistance to the nurse's aide, but you should communicate to the aide the importance of providing feedback on things observed and discussed while with the client. You could help the nurse's aide examine his or her thoughts about the client and take a therapeutic approach.

5. What criteria must be met for a diagnosis of Pain Disorder? Do this client's behaviors match the criteria? Fontaine and Fletcher (2003) make four points in regard to Pain Disorder:

1. The primary symptom of pain disorder is pain that does not lend itself to being explained organically.
2. The basis for this pain is thought to be unconscious conflict and anxiety.
3. The pain might disrupt a person's life.
4. Inadvertent substance abuse can occur.

The five criteria (APA, 2000; Frisch and Frisch, 2006) for a diagnosis of Pain Disorder involve:

1. Pain occurs in at least one anatomic location that is the major focus of clinical presentation and is severe enough to call for clinical attention.
2. Significant clinical distress or impaired social, occupational, and/ or other areas of the person's life result from the pain.

3. Psychological factors are believed to play a significant role in onset, duration, strength, and exacerbation of the pain.
4. There is no intentional production or feigning of the symptom or deficit.
5. If the person can meet the criteria for Somatization Disorder or if a mood, anxiety, or psychotic disorder better accounts for the pain, the diagnosis of Pain Disorder is not made.

The *Diagnostic and Statistical Manual of Mental Disorders* (APA, 2000) discusses sorting the diagnosis into either Pain Disorder Associated with Psychological Factors or Pain Disorder Associated with Both Psychological Factors and a General Medical Condition. The various areas of pain also can be coded and the duration can be specified as acute (less than six months) or chronic (more than six months).

Wanda's pain is chronic, as it has lasted longer than six months. She appears to meet all the criteria for chronic Pain Disorder, although nurses do not make this diagnosis. This client's pain is severe enough to call for clinical attention. There is impairment in occupational and social aspects of her life, as she lost her job and is separated from her husband and child. Whether her pain is associated with both psychological factors and a general medical condition or simply psychological factors is not necessarily important to the nurse. The nurse will treat the client with an open mind toward the possibility of a general medical condition, while looking for ways to assess and address psychological factors that are creating or adding to the client's problems.

6. How would you start to build a therapeutic relationship with Wanda? Ideas for building a therapeutic relationship would include responding quickly to her requests for pain medication, using a professional voice and manner, not promising anything that might prove undeliverable, talking to her as an adult, considering her part of the treatment team and problem solving together, and being interested in helping her find ways to deal with the physical pain and psychological distress.

7. What psychological stressors and cultural influences might have contributed to Wanda's chronic pain? Wanda came from a French Canadian culture, a culture in which people fear English diluting the culture and language, and put herself into an English culture. This movement away from familiar customs and friends and family was a stressor. Marrying was another stressor, as was attending message therapy school and having a child. Wanda's work was stressful, as she did not like speaking English to customers. Her relationship with her husband was a "love-hate relationship." Perhaps, subconsciously the headache pain provided Wanda a way to avoid dealing with this difficult relationship and other stressors. Because

Canadians have social medicine and access to inexpensive medical care, Wanda might have gone to the health care provider more frequently with her headache complaints. Although psychological stressors and cultural beliefs might have played a role in Wanda developing Pain Disorder, it might turn out that she has a medical problem. Thus, the nurse must keep an open mind about what causes and exacerbates Wanda's headaches.

8.   What nursing diagnoses would you write for this client? What would be some likely short-term goals for this client? Actual and possible diagnoses include:

- Pain
- Relocation stress syndrome
- Ineffective role performance (the client gave up performing the roles of wife, mother, and worker)
- Interrupted family processes
- Ineffective coping

Short-term goals might include:

- Identify two major stressors. The nurse can help the client begin to identify stressors by asking, "What things seem to worry you the most?"
- Identify at least one alternative or adjunct to pain medication for dealing with stress and/or pain (e.g., meditation, music, and massage).
- Establish contact with child's caregiver and child through a telephone call, written note, or other means.

9.   What nursing interventions would be helpful? Interventions could include finding someone who speaks French to talk with the client, or finding some music sung in French that would be relaxing. Other interventions could include teaching relaxation exercises, if the client is unfamiliar with these exercises; encouraging relaxation times, if the client is knowledgeable about relaxation; and positive reinforcement for all the activities in which the client engages such as showering, personal hygiene, and relaxation exercises. The nurse can offer a massage and/or facilitate the client's massage therapist coming to the hospital. In addition, the nurse can encourage the client to continue her meditation and help the client write a personal schedule that includes meditation time. The nurse could offer to help the client make telephone calls or provide writing materials to assist the client in reestablishing contact with her family and friends.

10. What are the current treatments for chronic Pain Disorder? A number of chronic pain rehabilitation clinics in the United States treat chronic pain originating in various parts of the body. Their approaches are usually holistic, utilizing techniques and tools such as group therapy, individual therapy, exercise, dietary changes, meditation, biofeedback, acupuncture, relaxation exercises, massage, physical therapy, music therapy, spiritual work, and other forms of therapy as well as a variety of medications and ways to deliver medications. A study (*Consumer Reports on Health*, 2004) on exercise's effect on neck pain found that the isometric exercise group had less pain after twelve months than groups doing endurance or aerobic exercises, while the endurance exercise group had less pain than the aerobics group.

Biofeedback is an effective treatment modality for migraine headaches and other chronic pain (Pulliam and Gatchel, 2003). Biofeedback helps the client develop awareness and some voluntary control over physiologic processes such as skin temperature, various brain wave rhythms, blood pressure, heart rate, and gastric motility.

Electroanalgesia, which involves the use of electric current, is used to control and manage pain. Most nurses are familiar with the transcutaneous electrical nerve stimulator (TENS) device. A newer system, the electronic nerve modulator (ENM), consists of self-adhesive pads that provide alternating positive and negative pulses. Use of electrical current to treat chronic pain is based on the gate theory of pain in which pain signals go up the spinal cord to the brain passing through a gate (*Journal of Therapy and Rehabilitation*, 2004).

The goal of treatment for chronic pain is to help clients cope with their pain, be functional, and resume their roles. As the treatment progresses, the client might experience less pain but often is not free of pain. Because the client is not totally focused on pain, she can focus on other responsibilities and activities of life.

Livingstone and Novak (2004) recommend an integrated headache reduction program (HARP) that involves support groups, breathing exercises, dietary changes, and other treatments including the latest medications. Novak (2004) underscores that migraines are commonly misperceived as a psychosomatic disorder arising from an inability to handle stress rather than a real disorder. She points out that most migraine sufferers have a family history of migraines, with 75–80 percent having a first-degree relative who also has disabling headaches. Migraine sufferers "have nervous systems that are unusually sensitive to environmental and internal factors: particularly light, odors, sound, hormonal fluctuations, weather changes, irregular sleep, certain foods, and skipped meals" (Novak, 2004). Novak also describes a physiologic basis for migraine onset—unstable neurotransmitter levels—and notes that migraine sufferers often have mood disorders, which occur via the same mechanism. Yerierski and associates (2004) say that chronic pain can cause anxiety, anger, and depression.

References

American Psychiatric Association (APA). (2000). *Diagnostic and Statistical Manual of Mental Disorders, 4th ed.* Text Revision. Washington, DC: American Psychiatric Association.

Fontaine, K. and K. Fletcher. (2003). *Mental Health Nursing.* Upper Saddle River, NJ: Pearson Education Inc.

Frisch, N. C. and L. E. Frisch. (2006). *Psychiatric Mental Health Nursing, 3d ed.* Albany, NY: Thomson Delmar Learning.

King, S. (2000). "The Classification and Assessment of Pain." 12: 86–90.

Livingstone, I. and D. Novak. (2004). *Breaking the Headache Cycle: A Proven Program for Treating and Preventing Recurring Headaches.* New York: Henry Holt and Company.

"A New Form of Electroanalgesia in the Management of Chronic Pain." (2004). *Journal of Therapy and Rehabilitation* 11(4): 146.

Novak, D. M. (February 2004). "Breaking the Headache Cycle." *Nursing Spectrum*, 1–9.

Pulliam. C. B., and R. J. Gatchel. (2002). "Biofeedback 2003: Its Role in Pain Management." *Journal of Internal Medicine* 17(3): 173–180.

"Special Strength Exercises Ease Neck Pain." (2004). *Consumer Reports on Health* 16(4): 10.

Spratto, G. R. and A. L. Woods. (2005). *2006 Edition PDR Nurses' Drug Handbook.* Clifton Park, NY: Thomson Delmar.

Yerierski, R. P., et al. (2004). *Nursing.* "Understanding Chronic Pain." 34(4): 22–24.

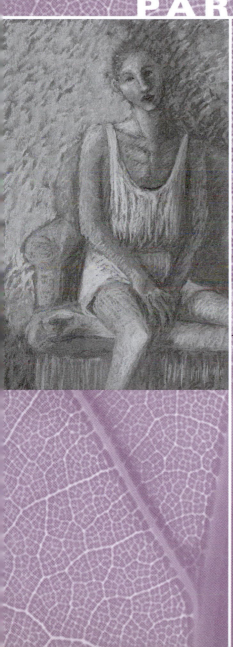

PART SEVEN

The Client with Disorders of Self-Regulation

Sam

GENDER

M

AGE

30

SETTING

- City public health clinic

ETHNICITY

- White American

CULTURAL CONSIDERATIONS

- Homeless

PREEXISTING CONDITION

COEXISTING CONDITION

COMMUNICATION

DISABILITY

SOCIOECONOMIC

SPIRITUAL/RELIGIOUS

PHARMACOLOGIC

PSYCHOSOCIAL

- Interactions limited to people he perceives as accepting him
- Alienated from family

LEGAL

- Prostitution is illegal
- Confidentiality must not be breached

ETHICAL

ALTERNATIVE THERAPY

PRIORITIZATION

DELEGATION

MODERATE

DISORDERS OF SELF-REGULATION

Level of difficulty: Moderate

Overview: Requires identification of thoughts and feelings about the client and critical thinking. The nurse must put aside personal feelings and adopt a professional therapeutic approach to the client. The nurse also must find health care and other needed resources for a homeless male client who wants to be a woman.

Client Profile

Sam is a 30-year-old homeless male. He sometimes sleeps in a wooded area with other homeless people, but more often finds a friend to stay with or a church shelter. Sam works off and on, but never enough to afford an apartment. Sam believes he is a woman and dresses in women's clothing, thus making it difficult to find steady employment. He is a tall, large-boned man with a deep, masculine voice. Even though he wears a wig and picks out nice clothing from a resale shop, people immediately recognize him as a man in women's clothing.

Sam has dressed in girls' clothing since he was a small child. At an early age, he played with dolls and preferred playing with girls. He has not had contact with his family of origin for years because they have difficulty accepting his behavior. He does call his mother from time to time, and she occasionally sends him a small check when he gives her an address.

Sam eats lunch nearly every weekday at a church dining room where a free meal is served to the homeless.

Case Study

The church parish nurse sees Sam, a big man dressed in women's clothing and wearing a wig and makeup. The nurse decides to find out more about his situation to see if she can help him in her role as parish nurse. The nurse offers Sam, and those around him, more coffee and introduces herself. Sam introduces himself as "Cindy." The seat next to Sam is empty, so the nurse sits down with a cup of coffee. Before long, Sam takes the nurse aside and begins to confide that he is getting hormone injections from a private doctor and free voice lessons from a voice coach at the nearby university. A week later, the nurse sees Sam at the church again; he says he is still taking voice lessons and hormone injections and looking forward to sex-change surgery some time. The nurse asks, "What worries you the most about these treatments?" She is surprised to hear him say, "I am worried most about paying for the treatments." Sam says that he pays with money earned from small jobs and by prostituting himself. He adds that he is concerned about contracting the human immunodeficiency virus (HIV). The nurse tells Sam about the city public health clinic. Sam promises to go there and be checked for HIV. He is willing to go because he hears that a former sexual partner is HIV positive.

Questions

1. What approach did the parish nurse use to build a therapeutic relationship with this client? What approach might you use?

2. What words or feelings come to mind as you think about approaching this client or one with similar behavior?

Questions (continued)

3. How would you address this client? Sam or Cindy?

4. Could this client be diagnosed as having Transvestic Fetishism? How well does this client match the criteria for diagnosis of Gender Identity Disorder (GID)?

5. What is the usual course of GID? What is its prevalence? What causes GID?

6. Was the nurse's question to Sam regarding his worst fear productive? Would you use this response or a different one?

7. Why didn't the nurse give the client a deadline for going to the city public health clinic?

8. If you were a nurse assisting with the physical examination of this client, would you see differences in the genitalia or other areas of the body?

9. Do all males with GID want to give up their penis for female genitalia?

10. In writing a care plan for a client with GID, what would you include in assessment, planning, implementation, and evaluation?

11. In what areas of nursing would a nurse have contact with clients who have GID?

Questions and Suggested Answers

1. What approach did the parish nurse use to build a therapeutic relationship with this client? What approach might you use? The parish nurse took a low-key approach, offering to refill coffee for the client and the people around him. She did not single the client out initially. She then offered her time and attention by sitting next to him. You could introduce yourself and share your role, saying something such as, "I am John, a student nurse helping serve lunch today. I would like to sit a few minutes with you." You want to begin building a relationship in a nonthreatening way. Another approach would be to ask the client to help you do some task after he is through eating. Being a help boasts a person's self-esteem and provides an opportunity to talk.

2. What words or feelings come to mind as you think about approaching this client or one with similar behavior? Your thoughts might vary from thinking the client is repulsive or sick to thinking he is fascinating or interesting. You can think or feel anything; however, you must put negative thoughts and feelings aside and adopt a positive attitude to work with the client. You may feel many different things such as revulsion, dislike, pity, desire to change the client to be more like you or to "fix" or rescue the client, or just feel you want to help the client.

If you have difficulty treating people equally or if you are prejudiced about homosexuality, transvestite behavior, or GID, you need to talk with your nursing supervisor. Because prejudices are learned, it is possible to unlearn them. Notably, homosexuality is not a diagnosis in the *Diagnostic and Statistical Manual of Mental Disorders* (APA, 2000). The American Psychiatric Association communicated in 1975 that homosexuality is not a disorder, and homophobia is prejudicial behavior often based in stereotypes. Like racism or sexism, homophobia can be unlearned (Tate and Longo, 2004).

3. How would you address this client? Sam or Cindy? You should use whatever name the client prefers, just as you would with any other client. To determine the client's preference, you should ask, "What name do you prefer to be called?" This client prefers the name "Cindy."

4. Could this client be diagnosed as having Transvestic Fetishism? How well does this client match the criteria for diagnosis of GID? Transvestic Fetishism involves a male cross-dressing in female attire and having sexual arousal produced by thoughts or images of self as a female. This disorder is quite different from wanting to be a woman.

Men with Transvestic Fetishism do not have a childhood history of cross-gender behaviors as children, except for possibly cross-dressing; although cross-dressing can begin in adulthood. The table below presents the diagnostic criteria for GID. Sam seems to fits this diagnosis.

Criteria for Diagnosis of GID	Do Client's Behaviors Match Diagnosis?
Strong, intense, lasting desire to be of another gender, or strong belief one is of another gender.	Yes, client has a long history of wanting to be female and thinking he is a female, beginning with cross-dressing and preferring to play with girls as a child.
Discomfort with own sex, or feeling inappropriate in gender role of that sex.	To be assessed.
A physical intersex condition is not concurrent with this concern.	This needs further assessment, but the condition does not appear to be due to partial androgen insensitivity syndrome or congenital adrenal hyperplasia.
The person experiences clinically significant impairment or distress in important areas of functioning such as social, occupational, or other areas.	Yes, the client can't get legitimate work due to the disorder and struggles as a prostitute, risking HIV infection and other health-altering consequences, in order to change sexual characteristics and possibly gender; the disorder narrows the client's social circle; and it alienates the client's family.

Adapted from the *Diagnostic and Statistical Manual of Mental Disorders* (APA, 2000).

5. What is the usual course of GID? What is its prevalence? What causes GID? Sometimes, but not always, GID is evident at a very early age. Parents might say their child has always had cross-gender behaviors. Parents tend to get more concerned when their child goes to school and his or her behavior is markedly different from his or her same-sex peers. It begins to cause the child distress when other children tease and taunt. Others with GID, particularly males, seem to start cross-gender behaviors in adolescence or early adulthood.

Perrin (2003) suggests that about 65 percent of boys diagnosed with GID will eventually embrace a gay lifestyle and 10 percent will be transgendered; some will eventually ask for sex reassignment through hormones and/or surgery. The remaining 25 percent will become heterosexual males. Bower (2000, 2) points out that about two-thirds of male-to-female transsexuals who are attracted to males "reject homosexual partners and desire virile, heterosexual males."

GID is more prevalent in males, by a ratio of some thirty to one. European data suggest one per thirty thousand men and one per one hundred thousand women seek sex-reassignment operations (APA, 2000).

The causes of GID are unknown. Manderson and Kumar (2001, 546) attribute the cause to a "psychological coping strategy in relation to trauma and abuse in childhood, and that the earlier the trauma occurs, the more rigid and unchanging the belief will be." If this is true, why do some people with traumatic childhoods develop GID while many more do not?

Another theory proposes biologic differences. There is a syndrome called Swyer syndrome in which babies are born with a male set of chromosomes and female genitalia. This syndrome involves the SRY protein, which is supposed to enter the nucleus of male gonadal cells in the fetus and turn on the genes that form the testes. In a somewhat complex mutation, the protein is unable to do so, and the fetus with male chromosomes does not develop male genitalia. This theory does not explain how this client is male and behaves female and wants to be female. It does open the door to thinking about biologic differences as a possible cause for GID (Sreenivasan, 2003).

6. Was the nurse's question to Sam regarding his worst fear productive? Would you use this response or a different one? The nurse's question is an open-ended question (i.e., not answerable with a yes or no), which produced some valuable information. In response, the client revealed his worry regarding paying for treatments, admitted to prostitution, and conveyed a fear about getting infected with a sexually transmitted disease. The nurse quickly learned what was on the client's mind. An opening of "What worries you the most about…?" is productive in other situations, such as when a client is discharged from an inpatient setting (e.g., "What worries you the most about going home?" or, in Sam's case, "What worries you the most about living on the street?"). There are many other responses you could use in this case.

7. Why didn't the nurse give the client a deadline for going to the city public health clinic? If she had added, "And I want you to promise to do this before you come to lunch here at the church next week," the client may resist thinking someone is trying to control him. A good reason not to give a deadline is, "What happens if the client misses the deadline?" If Sam doesn't go to the city public health clinic for any reason, he might decide he can't face the nurse. Then, the nurse loses the chance to try a different method to get the client to go to the clinic.

8. If you were a nurse assisting with the physical examination of this client, would you see differences in the genitalia or other areas of the body? People with GID almost always have normal genitalia for their gender unless they have had surgery to alter the genitalia. You might see enlarged breasts in male clients who have had hormone therapy. Some males have had thyroid cartilage shaving to reduce the size of their Adam's apple and body hair removed by various means.

Women with GID will sometimes be found on physical examination to be wearing a breast binder to flatten their breasts and occasionally will present with a skin rash from wearing it. Women also might be taking male hormones, such as testosterone enanthate injections, to deepen the voice and grow body hair.

9. Do all males with GID want to give up their penis for female genitalia? Not all males with GID want to give up their penis, as reported by Meyenburg (1999). Some males value their penis and only want face and neck surgery to look more female. Others might want breast enhancement but retain their penis.

10. In writing a care plan for a client with GID, what would you include in assessment, planning, implementation, and evaluation? You need to assess the client for suicidal ideation. This is a priority assessment and must be done on an ongoing basis. Since many clients with GID are, or later become, homosexual, this is important. It also is important because of the social stigma attached to any variation of the heterosexual orientation. McAndrew and Warner (2004, 428) state, "International epidemiological studies demonstrate that gay and bisexual males are four times more likely to report a serious suicide attempt than their heterosexual counterparts." In addition, it is helpful to assess the client's sexual orientation, which can fall under one of four categories: attracted to females, attracted to males, attracted to both sexes, or attracted to neither sex. Males with GID seem to fall into all the categories, while females almost always are attracted to females. About 66 percent of males who want transgender surgery are attracted to heterosexual males (Bower, 2000).

The nurse can assess the client's resources, including access to mental health counseling and services and supportive people or agencies. The nurse can help the client find additional resources, either personally or by referring the client to the community mental health center or a social worker. In assessing the client's resources, the nurse might look at the client's relationship with his family to determine if the client wants to improve this relationship and what the client thinks might help. The nurse can assess whether the client is isolating or not; if this is a problem, the nurse can work with the client to identify means for resolving this problem.

In looking at the client's shelter situation, the temptation is to find a place for the client to live without thoroughly assessing whether the client wants a permanent address or what type of living accommodations he wants. Some homeless people do not want an apartment or a room in a shared house. It is wise to remind yourself that everyone does not think about housing in the same way that you do.

If the client wants help finding a place to live, it is therapeutic to have him make some telephone calls and inquiries so he is invested in the process. This involvement will tend to make him more invested in the lifestyle change too.

The nurse needs to assess the client's high-risk sexual behavior and educate the client on taking precautions to avoid getting sexually transmitted diseases or not spreading sexually transmitted disease(s) to others.

The client's goal is to get hormone treatments and surgery to be more female. The nurse can listen to the client discuss this goal and help the client explore appropriate ways to meet it.

Evaluation will depend on what goals were set. One goal might be to stop prostitution and find appropriate ways to earn money to get the desired surgery. Another goal might be to identify and utilize two methods to reduce the risk of sexually transmitted diseases.

11. In what areas of nursing would a nurse have contact with clients who have GID? All nurses can expect to interact with a client who has GID at some time in their nursing career. These clients are seen in pediatric units, community clinics, schools, hospital medical and surgical units, plastic surgeons' offices, or endocrinologists' offices as well as every other medical, surgical, and mental health care area.

References

American Psychiatric Association (APA). (2000). *Diagnostic and Statistical Manual of Mental Disorders, 4th ed.* Text Revision. Washington, DC: American Psychiatric Association.

Bower, H. (2000). "The Gender Identity Disorder in the DSM-IV Classification: A Critical Evaluation." *Australian and New Zealand Journal of Psychiatry* 35(1): 1–8.

Manderson, L. and S. Kumar. (2001). "Gender Identity Disorder as a Rare Manifestation of Schizophrenia." *Australian and New Zealand Journal of Psychiatry* 55(4): 546–547.

McAndrew, S. and T. Warner. (2004). "Ignoring the Evidence Dictating the Practice: Sexual Orientation, Suicidality and the Dichotomy of the Mental Health Nurse." *Journal of Psychiatric Mental Health Nursing* 11(4): 428–434.

Meyenburg, B. (1999). "Gender Identity Disorder in Adolescence: Outcomes of Psychotherapy." *Adolescence* 34(134): 305–314.

Perrin, E. C. (2003). "Helping Parents and Children Understand 'Gender Identity Disorder.'" *Brown University Child and Adolescent Behavior Letter* 19(1): 1–4.

Sreenivasan, A. (2003). "Lockout Leads to Sex Reversal." *Science Now* 1216: 3.

Tate, F. B. and D. A. Longo. (2004). "Homophobia: A Challenge for Psychosocial Nursing." *Journal of Psychosocial Nursing and Mental Health Services* 42(8): 26–33.

CASE STUDY 2

Lily

GENDER

F

AGE

14

SETTING

- School Nurse

ETHNICITY

- Mexican American
  - Hispanic father
  - White American mother

CULTURAL CONSIDERATIONS

- American and Latino identification, with thin as beautiful

PREEXISTING CONDITION

COEXISTING CONDITION

COMMUNICATION

DISABILITY

SOCIOECONOMIC

- Middle-class, two-parent, working family

SPIRITUAL/RELIGIOUS

PHARMACOLOGIC

PSYCHOSOCIAL

LEGAL

ETHICAL

ALTERNATIVE THERAPY

PRIORITIZATION

DELEGATION

DISORDERS OF SELF-REGULATION

Level of difficulty: High

Overview: Requires knowledge of the client's culture and signs and symptoms of eating disorders, understanding of the developmental tasks of adolescence, critical thinking, and an open mind. The nurse must develop a workable plan of care and implement effective interventions that result in healthy eating behaviors.

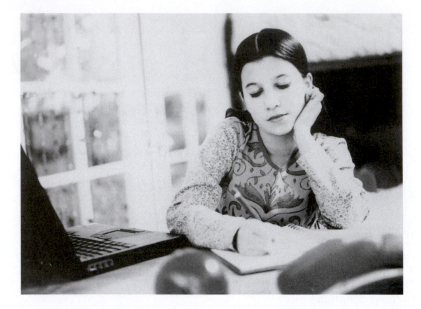

Client Profile

Lily is a 14-year-old high-school freshman from a middle-class family; both her parents work. Her father is Hispanic, and her mother is white American. She identifies with her father's Hispanic culture and idolizes the popular Latina singers.

Lily's teachers notice she is looking gaunt and appears to be underweight for her height. Lily is active and always "on the go." She is frequently seen running on the school track or in the neighborhood before school and at lunchtime. Her teachers comment about Lily's perfectionism; she recopies pages of work because her handwriting doesn't look as nice as it could or her paper has a flaw or a small ink smudge. A teacher monitoring the cafeteria sees Lily sitting by herself and observes her cutting her food into tiny pieces and pushing it from one area of her plate to another. She does not eat the food.

Case Study

Lily goes to the school nurse's office complaining of a stomachache. She tells the nurse that her period might be starting, as she has "missed three periods." She shares that she is normally irregular, and it is not unusual for her to miss one or two menstrual periods. The nurse takes Lily's vital signs and records the following data:

- Temperature: 96.8° F
- Pulse: 64
- Respirations: 12

Lily comments on being fat as the nurse weighs her and gets her height. Her height is 5 foot 6 inches and her weight is 96 pounds. The nurse tries to talk to Lily about being underweight for her height, but Lily persists in talking about being fat and how much her stomach sticks out. She draws a picture of herself: a picture that depicts a huge, protruding stomach. The nurse suspects that Lily has Anorexia Nervosa (AN). She starts to think of some way to talk to Lily's parents about what she has observed and the need for follow-up with their family health care provider.

Questions

1. What reason(s) could there be for this adolescent to miss menstrual periods? Discuss approaches the nurse might use to find out if the student is sexually active or not.

2. What are the essential features of Anorexia Nervosa? What signs or symptoms has the nurse observed that suggest Anorexia Nervosa? What additional signs and symptoms are seen in Anorexia Nervosa?

3. Are there different types of Anorexia Nervosa?

4. If you were the school nurse, what strategy would you use to talk to Lily's parents? What would you say to them?

5. If Lily is diagnosed with Anorexia Nervosa, how serious is this? What is the course of this disorder?

6. What are the current theories on the cause(s) of Anorexia Nervosa? Are there environmental and cultural factors in this case?

7. Would a school nurse ever observe or work with a male student with Anorexia Nervosa? If yes, what is the prevalence of Anorexia Nervosa in males compared to females?

8. Lily sees a health care provider who hospitalizes her for two weeks. When she returns to school, she goes to show the nurse a collection of recipes. She asks if she can be weighed every day. What do you think of this request? How would you respond if you were the school nurse?

9. How compliant are clients with Anorexia Nervosa? How likely is it that Lily will resist treatment for this condition?

10. What nursing diagnoses seem appropriate for Lily given what limited information you have? What approaches or interventions do you think would be good for the school nurse? How could the nurse utilize teachers and school resources to help this client?

11. What are some nonpharmacologic interventions used in the treatment of Anorexia Nervosa? Is medication helpful in treating Anorexia Nervosa? If so, what medications?

Questions and Suggested Answers

1. Why might this client miss menstrual periods? How could the nurse find out if Lily is sexually active? Discuss approaches the nurse might use to find out if the student is sexually active or not. If Lily has been sexually active, she could be pregnant; however, undernourishment and lack of body fat are more likely causes for her missed periods. Delayed onset of menses and/or missed menstrual periods is common in females who have malnutrition from any cause including Anorexia Nervosa.

The school nurse must use judgment about when and how to ask a student if she is sexually active. One approach would be to ask the student if she has any idea why she has missed three periods. Another nonthreatening means is to ask her a series of health questions, including one about whether or not the client is now sexually active or has ever been in the past.

2. What are the essential features of Anorexia Nervosa? What signs or symptoms has the nurse observed that suggest Anorexia Nervosa? What additional signs and symptoms are seen in Anorexia Nervosa? The essential features (APA, 2000) include:

- Refusal to maintain a minimally normal body weight (weight within 85 percent of expected weight for age and height)
- An intense fear of gaining weight
- Exhibition of significant disturbance in perception of size or shape of body
- Amenorrhea (defined as at least three missed menstrual cycles) in a post-menarchal female

The nurse observed that Lily is not within 85 percent of the normal weight for her age and height, but does not know the cause yet. The nurse needs to keep an open mind as to the cause. There are, however, other clues that Lily might have Anorexia Nervosa. Lily persists in saying she is fat, even though she is underweight. Individuals with Anorexia Nervosa seem to have an unconscious mental picture of an 89-pound ideal weight for themselves. Lily exhibits a disturbed perception of her body by drawing herself with a large stomach. She has missed three consecutive menstrual periods, which meets a diagnostic criterion for Anorexia Nervosa. In addition, the nurse has been told that Lily pushes food around on her plate but doesn't eat it. The nurse knows about her history of long, frequent jogs; this is a behavior consistent with someone trying to lose weight due to a fear of being too fat.

In AN, common symptoms include cold intolerance, constipation, decreased concentration, depression, fatigue, hair loss, and lightheadedness or dizziness. Common clinical signs include alopecia, bradycardia, cachexia, dry skin, hypotension, lanugo, peripheral edema, and stress fractures (Brubaker and Leddy, 2003). Lily has a slow pulse and a low temperature. The nurse needs to assess for additional signs and symptoms. Clients with Anorexia Nervosa who engage in binging and purging will eventually have parotid gland swelling and tooth enamel erosion.

Follow-up is essential, even for clients who don't meet all criteria for diagnosis. If this disorder is not treated early, it can be more difficult to treat later (Ressel, 2003). According to the American Academy of Pediatrics, more than half the children and adolescents with eating disorders do not fully meet the criteria in the diagnostic manual, but "still experience the same medical and psychological consequences of these illnesses" (Ressel, 2003, 205).

3. Are there different types of Anorexia Nervosa? There are two different types of Anorexia Nervosa: Restricting Type and Binge-Eating/Purging Type. In the Restricting Type, the client does not binge (i.e., eat more than a normal person would eat in a discrete period of time, usually less than two hours), self-induce vomiting, or abuse laxatives, diuretics, enemas, or other means to purge. In the Binge-Eating/Purging Type, the client engages in the preceding behaviors. The school nurse must gather data on whether Lily is binging and purging. This information could come from various sources (e.g., parents, siblings, peers).

4. If you were the school nurse, what strategy would you use to talk to Lily's parents? What would you say to them? It would likely be helpful for you to talk to each parent separately, as this encourages each one to talk freely. If possible, you would then meet with them together to provide some idea of the dynamics of the couple. If the parents want to meet with you together first, you have the option to schedule separate follow-up meetings with each parent later.

You must listen and gently probe to find out what the parents' perceptions of Lily are and whether or not they perceive that she has a problem with food and weight. You should communicate a caring attitude toward Lily and project a desire to work with them to help Lily be in the best health possible. In talking with the parents, you might decide not to bring up the idea of a possible eating disorder if they give cues they are unreceptive to this possibility. In some cases, parents are in denial; they will react with extreme anger and withdraw their child from the school system. If you sense denial on the part of the parents, you should refer them to their pediatrician or family health care provider to look into the missed menstrual periods. You need to get the parents to sign a release of information form in order to share information with the pediatrician or family health care provider.

It is possible that Lily has already been diagnosed and is under the care of a professional who specializes in eating disorders. The parents might have just failed to communicate this information to the school.

5. If Lily is diagnosed with Anorexia Nervosa, how serious is this? What is the course of this disorder? Anorexia Nervosa is a serious disorder with the potential to be fatal. About 5.6 percent of persons with Anorexia Nervosa die each year. The long-term mortality is estimated at over 10%, with death resulting from complications such as electrolyte imbalance, starvation, or suicide associated with the disorder (APA, 2000).

Palmer (2004) and the *Harvard Mental Health Letter* (2003) suggest that Anorexia Nervosa might not be as deadly as previously thought. Both cite the Korndorfer Study at the Mayo Clinic, which looked at 208 cases of Anorexia Nervosa over a 55-year period and found no excessive mortality rates. Nurses still need to keep in mind that clients can and do die from complications of Anorexia Nervosa.

Persons with malnutrition associated with Anorexia Nervosa can develop hyponatremia or hypernatremia from drinking too little or too much water to manipulate their weight. Cardiac dysrhythmias can result from electrolyte imbalance. Clients often have abdominal pain, gastrointestinal distress, bloating with meals, delayed gastric emptying, and constipation. Persons with Anorexia Nervosa often have a hard time concentrating. Malnutrition usually results in menstrual dysfunction with most females having amenorrhea. Amenorrhea can result in a long-term complication of osteopenia and later osteoporosis. Organ systems can fail in severe malnutrition (e.g., the client can experience kidney failure) (Resell, 2003).

6. What are the current theories on the cause(s) of Anorexia Nervosa? Are there environmental and cultural factors affecting this case? There is no current agreement on the cause of Anorexia Nervosa. An older theory suggests this disorder develops from a desire to avoid adult sexual development and responsibility. A more contemporary theory views it as a developmental disorder arising from disorganized family dynamics. People with Anorexia Nervosa often have a strong need for control and a tendency toward perfectionism. Thus, some theorists speculate that when persons fail to achieve the control they need or want in various aspects of their life, they will try to gain control over eating and weight. Family systems theorists suggest a family structure with marital discord, emphasis on control, and overprotectiveness as a causative factor. Some family theorists suggest that family dynamics are not causative but serve to enable the disorder as the family becomes enmeshed with poor boundaries and everyone in the family becomes preoccupied with food and eating rituals.

Another theory is American society's obsession with thin as beautiful, as fueled by the media. The influence of the parents on a child's body image and parental messages to diet might be factors in development of eating disorders. Body image dissatisfaction can start as early as age 5 (Coughlin et al., 2003).

Jilek (2001, 1) points out, "In North America the incidence of Anorexia Nervosa increased dramatically since the 1960s, coinciding with a drastic change in the feminine body ideal towards thinness." He also points out that weight tables used by American health care providers to provide normal standards moved downward in female body normals as the cultural ideal moved downward. Jilek states that since the 1960s, cases of Anorexia Nervosa have increased in non-Western areas such as Japan and Hong Kong because of Westernizing influences. Brubaker and Leddy (2003, 15) state, "While the exact prevalence is unknown, studies suggest that 15–62 percent of female athletes may struggle with disordered eating and male athletes are also affected." Examples of male athletes who might go overboard in weight loss are wrestlers wanting to be in a lighter weight class or runners who believe that weight slows them down.

Blinder and associates (1988) discuss the possibility that the homosexual culture possibly places a male at greater risk for Anorexia Nervosa because of the cultural pressure for homosexual males to be thin and attractive.

In Lily's case, culture might play a role. The Hispanic cultures—and the Latina singers she admires—are adopting the American ideal of thinness as a desired trait. An article in *Women's Health Weekly* (2003) says that many Hispanic women are critical of their bodies and are feeling the pressure to be thin. This article describes a study that found that Hispanic girls are more likely to report the most frequent weight loss attempts over the previous year and the highest number of binge-eating episodes.

Although cultural influences in the development of Anorexia Nervosa seem clear, could the cause be genetic? Anorexia Nervosa often is found in more than one family member, and studies in the past ten years suggest genes play a role. While the risk for an eating disorder is about half a percent in the general population, researchers found it to increase to elevenfold in persons who have relatives with Anorexia Nervosa (Backman, 2003). The National Alliance on Mental Illness (NAMI, 2003) states that if a girl has a sibling with Anorexia Nervosa, she has ten to twenty times higher risk for developing the disease compared to a girl without a family member with the disease. Research has found two genes that have sequence variations in anorexic women: "One of the gene codes for a protein that allows neurons to respond to serotonin, a neurotransmitter involved in mood. The other gene code is for an opioid receptor, which, among other things, is involved in appetite" (Backman, 2003, 3).

Perhaps Anorexia Nervosa is caused by a combination of psychological, cultural, family, developmental, and biologic factors (Kitsantas et al., 2003). Perhaps some cases of Anorexia Nervosa are more genetically based while others are more the result of cultural influences and learned behaviors. The bottom line is that there is no agreement at this time on the exact cause of this disorder.

7.   Would a school nurse ever observe or work with a male student with Anorexia Nervosa? If yes, what is the prevalence of Anorexia Nervosa in males compared to females? A school nurse could observe or work with a male student who has Anorexia Nervosa. The prevalence of males in the eating disorder population is said to be about 10 percent of all cases; some researchers feel this percentage is growing (Kerr-Price and Fowler, 2003). NAMI (2003) points out that conservatively 0.5–1 percent of females in the United States develop Anorexia Nervosa. Because 90 percent of all cases involve adolescent young women, it is thought to be a women's disease. However, males and children as young as seven have been diagnosed, as have women as old age 80. Blinder and colleagues (1988) state that Anorexia Nervosa has been diagnosed in children as young as age 4.

8.   Lily sees a health care provider who hospitalizes her for two weeks. When she returns to school, she goes to show the nurse a collection of recipes. She asks if she can be weighed every day. What do you think of this request? How would you respond if you were the school nurse? This request might be indicative of poor progress in treatment. People with Anorexia Nervosa can collect recipes, talk about foods to eat, cook and serve food to others, and still be losing weight from not eating. Although proof of progress lies in weight gain, the client's preoccupation with weight may be indicative of continued desire to weigh less rather than more. If the client is under treatment for Anorexia Nervosa, the treatment team might have set a schedule for weighing. Often, the treatment team will weigh the client standing backward on the scale to prevent the client from seeing the weight. These procedures take the focus off of weight. Before agreeing to weigh the client daily, the nurse needs to check with the client's treatment provider.

9.   How compliant are clients with Anorexia Nervosa? How likely is it that Lily will resist treatment for this condition? What developmental stage is this client in and does this relate to the degree of compliance in any way? Kaplan (2004) suggests that clients with Anorexia Nervosa often do not want to be treated and resist treatment. They are successful in deceiving parents, nurses, health care providers, and mental health care professionals in regard to their eating behaviors. Some people want to hold on to their disorder and encourage others to do so as well. They are part of a pro-anorexia movement ("Oprah Winfrey Show," 2005). Parents and health professionals working with children and adolescents with Anorexia Nervosa need to be aware of these websites (e.g., http://www.plagueangel.net/grotto) and deny access to them.

Lily falls into Erickson's adolescent stage (age 12–19) in which the developmental task is identity versus role confusion. The tasks of this stage include beginning to separate from parents, forming an identity, mastering independence, and forming relationships with the opposite gender. Clients of any age with Anorexia Nervosa are resistant to treatment; however, an adolescent might be more resistant because she is trying to separate from her parents and has different ideas than her parents. Working collaboratively with other team members will be important in helping this client meet the tasks of this stage of development and master her disorder.

10. What nursing diagnoses seem appropriate for Lily given what limited information you have? What approaches or interventions do you think would be good for the school nurse? How could the nurse utilize teachers and school resources to help this client? Appropriate nursing diagnoses include: Imbalanced nutrition: less than body requirements; Chronic low self-esteem; Disturbed body image; and Ineffective health maintenance. Further assessment might lead to a nursing diagnosis of Social isolation. An adolescent with an eating disorder might socially isolate for many reasons including feeling she is too fat and too ugly to be accepted by others and/ or being too busy with behaviors to lose weight to associate with others.

Further assessment might support a nursing diagnosis of Altered family processes, Anxiety, related to fears of gaining weight, and/or Powerlessness, related to lack of control.

The school nurse must follow school policies in alerting the school psychologist and school administration to the situation, including them as part of the school "team" working with this family. Initially, building rapport and trust with the family is an essential intervention. With rapport and trust, the nurse can educate the family about eating disorders and the importance of getting early treatment for an eating disorder, or behavior that might lead to an eating disorder, to prevent serious health problems. The nurse can discuss with the parents how their choice of communication and behaviors related to eating, weight, and body image might affect Lily positively or negatively and encourage healthy communication and behavior.

The school nurse can provide educational materials on eating disorders to the teachers and lead discussion groups on this topic with them. Teachers have many opportunities to set up self-esteem-building situations and help students tie their self-esteem to skills, talents, and performance rather than body image. Teachers can devise situations to help socially isolated students interact with their peers. In this case, the school nurse can work with Lily's teachers and help them identify ways to help her improve her self-esteem and body image and interact with her peers.

The nurse can continue to encourage teachers and provide positive reinforcement for appropriate work with Lily. With a signed consent from the parents, the nurse can work with any treatment providers that Lily and her family are consulting and ensure that approaches at school are helpful and consistent with those outside the school. The nurse can ensure that the school administration, school psychologist, and teachers are informed and involved, as appropriate or prescribed by policy.

11. What are some nonpharmacologic interventions used in the treatment of Anorexia Nervosa? Is medication helpful in treating Anorexia Nervosa? If so, what medications? When the client is severely malnourished, the problem of imbalanced nutrition is the priority and the client is usually hospitalized. The treatment team will focus on getting the client to take in more calories and preventing any client efforts to lose weight such as excessive exercise, use of laxatives, and self-induced vomiting. Clients might contract to eat a reasonable amount (e.g., 1,000 to 1,500 calories a day or 50–75 percent of the meals served on a prescribed number of calories diet). Instead of calories or percentage of meals eaten, the treatment goal might be a weight gain of 0.1 to 0.2 kg/day until the target weight is reached (White, 2000). Treatment teams sometimes have children or adolescents eat in a group and offer distractions during the meal to take the focus off of eating or not eating. Supervised dining also helps prevent the hiding, disposing, or flushing away of food. Conversation is not to focus on what to eat, how much to eat, begging or bribing for eating. When clients do not eat and are severely undernourished, they are sometimes fed by enteral feedings or total parental nutrition. This is not to be conveyed as a punishment but rather simply a consequence of not eating in a healthy manner. Denial of requests to go on unit outings or to be discharged home are also logical consequence of not eating.

When the client is eating appropriately and gaining weight, the focus of treatment starts to include interventions focused on dealing with psychosocial problems. Individual, group, and family therapy are often begun in the hospital phase and continued on an outpatient basis after discharge. In family therapy, the family is often encouraged to let the client take responsibility for his or her intake of food and fluids. In group therapy, clients with Anorexia Nervosa, who are very perfectionistic, might be assigned a task to do something imperfect.

Treatment programs often include instruction on ways to reduce stress and to relax as well as assertiveness training. A number of treatment programs focus not only on the attainment of a weight in the normal range, but also an acceptance of that weight. Some programs use photographs and/or videotapes of a client side by side with another person to help the client recognize how thin he or she is.

The role of the nurse in working with clients with Anorexia Nervosa includes being a role model of healthy eating, exercise, and recreational diversions. The role of the nurse also includes limit setting and education. Often a multidisciplinary team approach is used to manage various aspects of treatment (e.g., a health care provider for medical aspects, a psychiatrist to manage any psychotropic medications and/or the psychiatric aspects, a psychologist for testing, a master's-trained therapist for group and individual therapies, a registered dietitian, and nurses to provide nursing care and assist in the management of the milieu twenty-four hours a day and seven days a week).

Inpatient programs often use a level system wherein a client attains a higher level with more privileges for reaching each goal. Children and adolescents often do well with this system as they find they are not allowed to participate in activities until they take in the nourishment they need (Kerr-Price and Fowler, 2003).

Some programs use hypnosis to augment treatment. Mantle (2003) points out that some feel that these clients are poor subjects for hypnosis; however, hypnosis is helpful in facilitating the reduction of anxiety, conflict resolution, and coping strategies, as well as for rehearsing healthy self-talk, safe place imagery, and ways to deal with social phobia. Hypnosis also is used for age regression to uncover origins of possible cognitive distortions and emotional conflicts.

Cognitive restructuring, as described by Burns (1999) as a drug-free treatment for depression, also is used in work with clients with Anorexia Nervosa. These clients often use cognitive distortions and frequently suffer from depression.

Brubaker and Leddy (2003) describe five principles in effective treatment:

1. Allow time for the development of a therapeutic relationship.
2. Involve the client in the development of the contract.
3. Include appropriate outcome and process goals in the contract.
4. Provide a mechanism for monitoring progress toward contracted goals.
5. Carry out consequences with consistency.

The role of medication in treating children and adolescents with AN is not well explored (Muscari, 2002). Lithium carbonate (Eskalith, Lithobid), antidepressants, and some atypical antipsychotics might help. Brewerton (2004, 59) states that food is the drug of choice for clients with Anorexia Nervosa, and no drug "has been shown in double-blind, placebo-controlled trials to significantly improve Anorexia Nervosa when given outside a structured inpatient program."

References

American Psychiatric Association (APA). (2000). *Diagnostic and Statistical Manual of Mental Disorders, 4th ed.* Text Revision. Washington, DC: American Psychiatric Association.

Backman, M. (2003). "How Eating Disorders Are Inherited. *Science Now*, 3.

Blinder, B. J., et al., eds. (1988). *The Eating Disorders: Medical and Psychological Bases of Diagnosis and Treatment, 2d ed.* New York: PMA Publishing.

Brewerton, T. D. (2004). "Pharmacotherapy for Patients with Eating Disorders." Psychiatric Times 21(6): 59–61.

Brubaker, D. A. and J. J. Leddy. (2003). "Behavioral Contracting in the Treatment of Eating Disorders." Physician and Sports Medicine 31(9): 15–18.

Burns, D. D. (1999). Feeling Good: The New Mood Therapy. New York: New American Library.

Coughlin, J. W., et al. (2003). "Body Image Dissatisfaction in Children: Prevalence and Parental Influence." Healthy Weight Journal 17(40): 56–60.

"Eating Disorders Among U.S. Hispanic Women Are Up." (July 31, 2003). Women's Health Weekly, 61.

"In Brief—Anorexia: Not So Deadly."(2003). Harvard Mental Health Letter 20(2).

Jilek, W. G. (2001). "Cultural Factors in Psychiatric Disorders." www.mentalhealth.com/mag1/wolfgang.html. Accessed June 13, 2006.

Kaplan, A. (2004). "Treating Eating Disorders: The Pitfalls and Perplexities." Psychiatric Times 21(9): 4–5.

Kerr-Price, N., and K. Fowler. (2003). "Treating Kids with Eating Disorders." Behavioral Health Management 23(6): 28–33.

Kitsantas, A, et al. (2003). "College Women with Eating Disorders: Self-Regulation, Life Satisfaction, and Positive/Negative Affect." Journal of Psychology 137(4): 381–395.

Mantle, F. (2003). "Eating Disorders: The Role of Hypnosis." Paediatric Nursing 15(7): 42–45.

Muscari, M. (2002). "Effective Management of Adolescents with Anorexia and Bulimia." Journal of Psychosocial Nursing 40(2): 23–31.

National Alliance on Mental Awareness. (2003). "Anorexia Nervosa." www.nami.org/helpline/anorexia.htm. Accessed June 13, 2006.

"Oprah Winfrey Show." (2005). "Pro-Anorexia on the Web." www.oprah.com/tows/pastshows/tows_past_20011004_c.jhtml. Accessed June 13, 2006.

Palmer, R. L. (2003). "Death in Anorexia Nervosa." Lancet 361(9368): 1490.

Ressel, G. W. (2003). "AAP Releases Policy Statements on Identifying and Treating Eating Disorders." American Family Physician 67(10): 2224–2226.

White, L. (2000). Foundations of Nursing: Caring for the Whole Person. Albany, NY: Thomson Delmar Learning.

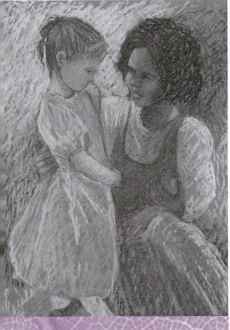

PART EIGHT

Special Populations: The Child, Adolescent, or Elderly Client

CASE STUDY 1

Tanya

GENDER

F

AGE

17

SETTING

- Obstetrician's office

ETHNICITY

- Black American

CULTURAL CONSIDERATIONS

- Southern
- Black American
- Eating nonnutritive substances could be a culturally sanctioned practice

PREEXISTING CONDITION

COEXISTING CONDITION

COMMUNICATION

DISABILITY

SOCIOECONOMIC

SPIRITUAL/RELIGIOUS

PHARMACOLOGIC

PSYCHOSOCIAL

LEGAL

ETHICAL

- Client's right to eat what she chooses against needs of unborn child

ALTERNATIVE THERAPY

PRIORITIZATION

DELEGATION

MODERATE

SPECIAL POPULATIONS: THE CHILD, ADOLESCENT, OR ELDERLY CLIENT

Level of difficulty: Moderate

Overview: Requires the use of therapeutic communication skills, critical thinking, and collaboration. The nurse must determine if the client has Pica and, if so, gather data about family history and interpret these data. The nurse must build a trusting relationship with the client's boyfriend and enlist his help in getting the client to follow a nutritive diet. The nurse also must work with other health care professionals and identify resources to assist the client.

Client Profile

Tanya is a 17-year-old pregnant female (twenty-two weeks' gestation) who lives with her mother. Her family has lived in the South for several generations. Her boyfriend, who is the baby's father, attends high school; Tanya dropped out of high school. In her first trimester, Tanya experienced some nausea and vomiting and did not gain any weight. She is not eating much.

Case Study

Tanya comes to the obstetrician's office for a routine prenatal check-up with her aunt. The aunt shares that Tanya's boyfriend is at school and her mother is at work. The office nurse remembers Tanya from previous visits to the office. At the last visit, the obstetrician was concerned because Tanya's had lost weight. When the nurse goes to the waiting room to get Tanya, she sees that the client is eating a large cup of shaved ice; a small cooler is nearby.

The nurse weighs Tanya. She now weighs a pound less than at her previous visit. Her vital signs are

- Blood pressure: 134/88 mm Hg
- Pulse: 92
- Respirations: 22

The nurse spends a few minutes talking with Tanya about clothing styles, saying how nice she looks. The nurse comments, "I notice you brought a little cooler with you." Tanya replies: "It's for ice. I have such a craving for ice." The nurse wants to know how much ice Tanya is consuming each day and what kind of ice it is. She also wants to know about any other "cravings." The nurse considers which therapeutic communication technique to use.

The laboratory technician enters the examination room to draw blood for a hemoglobin and hematocrit. The nurse leaves for a few minutes; when she returns, she notices some white substance on Tanya's lips. The nurse observes, "I notice you have something white on your lips." Tanya responds, "I just ate a little bit of starch." The nurse shares the findings of the nursing assessment and her observations regarding the client with the obstetrician. They both agree that the nurse should talk to the aunt about any family members who might have the habit of eating nonnutritive substances when pregnant or at other times, as well as Tanya's habits.

After the obstetrician examines Tanya, she asks the nurse to call the laboratory for the hemoglobin and hematocrit results. The laboratory report is:

- Hemoglobin: 10.8
- Hematocrit: 31%

The nurse learns from the aunt that one of Tanya's brothers began eating foam stuffing from the sofa and other sources when he was about 5 years old.

The obstetrician talks with Tanya and her aunt about the possibility of Tanya's boyfriend accompanying them on Tanya's next appointment.

Questions

1. What is the most likely explanation for Tanya's weight loss?

2. How does the nurse try to establish rapport with the client and her aunt? If you were the nurse in this case, how would you establish rapport with the client, the aunt, and the boyfriend?

3. If you were the nurse, how would you ask the client about the ice and starch that she is eating? Why would you be interested in this information?

4. How would you interpret the hemoglobin and hematocrit report?

5. Why would the obstetrician ask about the possibility of Tanya's boyfriend coming on her next visit?

6. What influence might the client's culture have on her life? How would you relate to this client to learn more about her culture?

7. Why is the nurse interested in non-nutritive eating habits within Tanya's family?

8. Does Tanya meet the diagnostic criteria for Pica? Does her brother meet these criteria?

9. What groups of people engage in Pica behaviors? What is the current thinking about the etiology of Pica?

10. What nursing diagnoses and goals would you most likely write for this client? What nursing interventions would be helpful for this client?

Questions and Suggested Answers

1. What is the most likely explanation for Tanya's weight loss? The client is most likely losing weight because she feels full after eating the non-nutritive ice and the noncaloric starch substance. Eating ice also might diminish feelings of hunger and satisfy the need to chew. Eating small amounts of ice is not unusual; however, this client is carrying around a small ice chest.

2. How does the nurse try to establish rapport with the client and her aunt? If you were the nurse in this case, how would you establish rapport with the client, the aunt, and the boyfriend? The nurse talks with the client about clothing styles, a topic of interest to adolescent girls. She also tells Tanya how nice she looks, probably in an effort to put her at ease. The nurse also uses some therapeutic techniques, including observation: "I notice you have brought a little cooler with you." and "I notice you have something white on your lips." The nurse avoids accusing the client or jumping to any conclusions. Her statements serve as an invitation to the client to explain in her own words.

As the nurse in this case, you would want to select a nonthreatening topic to begin building trust and rapport. You would talk to the client as an adult and treat her in a respectful manner. You should solicit her opinions and respect them. You should use language she can understand, but still use medical terms, at times, with a simple explanation to build the client's vocabulary and understanding of the terms health care professionals will be using as she progresses through pregnancy and delivery.

3. If you were the nurse, how would you ask the client about the ice and starch that she is eating? Why would you be interested in this information? You need to be gentle in your approach, using a nonthreatening, soft, matter-of-fact voice. You should use open-ended questions and employ encouraging statements such as "Go on" or "Tell me more about that." You want to find out if the client is eating any other non-nutritive substances because this behavior can put the fetus at risk of not receiving enough nutrients. In addition to insufficient nutrition, the client might be exposing the fetus to environmental toxins. This client is at risk for anemia and possibly constipation.

4. How would you interpret the hemoglobin and hematocrit report? The normal female hemoglobin is 12–16 g/dL, and the normal hematocrit is 37–47 percent. This client's hemoglobin is 10.8 and her hematocrit is 31 percent. These low values suggest iron deficiency anemia. The health care team should look for any and all causes, the most obvious of which are Pica and the extra demand placed on the body by the fetus.

5. Why would the obstetrician ask about the possibility of Tanya's boyfriend coming on her next visit? The obstetrician wants to determine what role the boyfriend will play in the prenatal, labor, and post-delivery periods as well as what role Tanya and her aunt will allow him to take. The nurse also wants to talk with them collectively to devise a plan to help Tanya gain weight and improve her prenatal condition. The nurse certainly wants to educate everyone who has an influence on what Tanya eats, or does not eat, about how to support her in decreasing nonnutritive substances and increasing nutritive ones.

6. What influence might the client's culture have on her life? How would you relate to this client to learn more about her culture? Some researchers report that Pica is found all over the world, and in the United States, it is more commonly found in Southern women, particularly rural black women, and those from a specific region of the state of Georgia (Smulian and Motiwala, 1995; Griggsby et al., 1999). In some cultures, children are fed nonnutritive substances such as starch or kaolin as a pacifier; some women engage in eating nonnutritive substances because older role models do so. Some cultures believe that certain substances are beneficial to the growing fetus. Likewise, Tanya's culture might influence decisions on the role the baby's father will play in the baby and mother's lives, whether the client will return to high school, and whether social services will be accessed. The nurse must keep an open mind because the black culture is changing, and differences exist among various subsets of blacks.

As the nurse, you need to relate to this client in an open-minded, nonjudgmental way, encouraging her to talk about her values and beliefs and thoughts about diet, pregnancy, and nutrition.

7. Why is the nurse interested in nonnutritive eating habits within Tanya's family? Eating foam-rubber stuffing from a sofa or other sources is sometimes found in children and adolescents with sickle cell anemia. Whether Tanya's brother has sickle cell anemia or not, he is eating a nonnutritive substance. The brother needs to have further evaluation in regard to his nutritional state and to determine any symptoms of sickle cell anemia which would warrant follow up. Lemanek and associates (2002, 493) conducted a study of the "incidence and relationship of pica symptoms and dysfunctional eating patterns in children and adolescents with sickle cell disease" and found subjects with and without symptoms of Pica who had dysfunctional eating patterns.

8. Does Tanya meet the diagnostic criteria for Pica? Does her brother meet these criteria? For a person to be diagnosed with Pica, the client must be persistently eating at least one and possibly more nonnutritive substances for at least a month. This behavior must not be part of a culturally sanctioned practice, and it must be developmentally inappropriate. If the person has a mental disorder and the eating of a nonnutritive substance occurs only during the course of this mental disorder, Pica is not diagnosed unless the eating of the substance is severe enough to warrant separate clinical attention.

At this point you do not have enough information to determine if the client or her brother can meet a diagnosis of Pica. The client has been eating at least two nonnutritive substances for over a month: ice and starch. This is not developmentally appropriate behavior at this stage in the client's life. The eating of starch could be a culturally sanctioned practice and this needs further assessment. The eating of ice and starch is at the point it warrants separate clinical attention because she is not gaining sufficient weight with her pregnancy and her hemoglobin and hematocrit are low.

9. What groups of people engage in Pica behaviors? What is the current thinking about the etiology of Pica? Pica is most often diagnosed in childhood or adolescence, although it can occur in infancy. The materials most often ingested include paint, plaster, cloth, hair, and string. Older children have been found to eat sand, insects, leaves, and pebbles, while adolescents and adults eat clay or soil as well as ashes and ice. Hackworth and Williams (2003) report on three cases of Pica involving foam rubber among the sickle cell disease population. All three cases involved black American males (one age 15 and the other two age 11). These researchers point out "reports from other researchers also suggest that this is not an uncommon form of pica" (Hackworth and Williams, 2003, 81).

Smulian and Motiwala (1995) report that pregnant women sometimes eat large amounts of ice, including freezer frost scraped from the freezer, cornstarch, laundry starch, soap, paint, burnt matches, and various types of earth, including kaolin. Their study found 18 of 125 pregnant rural women from Muscogee County, Georgia, had Pica behavior. About half of these subjects engaged in Pica behaviors when not pregnant, and a third had engaged in these behaviors as children.

Kaolin is also known as white clay, chalk, or white dirt. Grigsby and colleagues (1999, 192) found that kaolin ingestion "is primarily practiced by black women who were introduced to the behavior by family members or friends, either as children or during pregnancy." They did not find it to be a widespread practice among black American women, but that 14.4 percent of pregnant women from a rural area in Georgia exhibited some Pica behavior. These authors conclude that kaolin ingestion seems to meet the *Diagnostic and Statistical Manual of Mental Disorders* (APA, 2000) criteria for a "culture bound syndrome." In other words, these women have Pica behavior but do not meet the diagnostic criteria for a diagnosis of Pica since their behavior is culturally sanctioned. Smulian and Motiwala (1995) cite other reports of culturally sanctioned Pica. One, a report by Bruhn and Pangborn on pregnant migrant women of Mexican or Anglo descent, indicated these women ate cigarette ashes, clay pots, magnesia de tierra (magnesium carbonate), adobe, or tobacco.

Four etiologic theories of causation exist: psychological, pharmacologic, cultural, and nutritional. The theories seem to overlap. Some people with Pica feel it is beneficial in various ways such as making the baby stronger, better in color, or without birthmarks. Some cultures use nonnutritive substances as a pacifier for an infant. Hawkworth and Williams (2003, 83) question whether Pica could be an attempt to remedy some deficiency in the body, or not, and point out that other researchers have "discussed Pica in the context of obsessive-compulsive disorders in general."

10. What nursing diagnoses and goals would you most likely write for this client? What nursing interventions would be helpful for this client? Based on existing assessment findings, you would write nursing diagnosis of Imbalanced Nutrition: Less Than Body Requirements. After assessing the client for problems of elimination, you might find a problem with constipation. You then could write a nursing diagnosis of Constipation or At Risk for Constipation, depending on what you found. Another possible diagnosis is Fatigue, as pregnancy often brings fatigue; low hemoglobin and hematocrit values indicate less oxygen is being carried to cells and implies fatigue. Additional nursing diagnoses could include Disturbed Body Image, Situational Low Self-Esteem, and Knowledge Deficit about such things as pregnancy, childcare, and nutrition.

Interventions will be based on the nursing diagnoses. This client likely needs some prenatal vitamins with iron and education about nutrition. In addition, the nurse should discuss the importance of prenatal care, including rest, exercise, and nutrition.

References

American Psychiatric Association (APA). (2000). *Diagnostic and Statistical Manual of Mental Disorders, 4th ed.* Text Revision. Washington, DC: American Psychiatric Association.

Grigsby, R. K., et al. (1999). "Chalk Eating in Middle Georgia: A Culture-Bound Syndrome of Pica?" *Southern Medical Journal* 92: 190–194.

Hackworth, S. R. and L. L. Williams. (2003). "Pica for Foam Rubber in Patients with Sickle Cell Anemia." *Southern Medical Journal* 96: 81–84.

Lemanek, K. L. (2002). "Dysfunctional Eating Patterns and Symptoms of Pica in Children and Adolescents with Sickle Cell Disease." *Clinical Pediatrics* 41: 493–500.

Smulian, J. C. and S. Motiwala. (1995). "Pica in a Rural Obstetrical Population." *Southern Medical Journal* 88(12): 1236–1241.

CASE STUDY 2

Luke

GENDER

M

AGE

10

SETTING

- Infirmary of church summer day camp

ETHNICITY

- White American

CULTURAL CONSIDERATIONS

- Fundamentalist religion

PREEXISTING CONDITION

- Attention Deficit Hyperactivity Disorder (ADHD)

COEXISTING CONDITION

COMMUNICATION

- Requires one instruction at a time due to ADHD

DISABILITY

SOCIOECONOMIC

- Middle class

SPIRITUAL/RELIGIOUS

- Fundamentalist church

PHARMACOLOGIC

- Nystatin (Mycostatin)

PSYCHOSOCIAL

- Family activities, which revolve around church, are serious
- Need for play and relaxation in the family

LEGAL

- Child and Family Services threatens to take client away from family if the father does not use appropriate discipline

ETHICAL

ALTERNATIVE THERAPY

- Prayer
- Diet free of yeast products

PRIORITIZATION

DELEGATION

MODERATE

SPECIAL POPULATIONS: THE CHILD, ADOLESCENT, OR ELDERLY CLIENT

Level of difficulty: Moderate

Overview: Requires an understanding of the behaviors of children who have Tourette's Disorder, especially those demonstrated by this client. The nurse must identify approaches that hold promise for reducing disruptive behaviors and approaches that should be avoided.

Client Profile

Luke is a 10-year-old boy who was diagnosed with Attention Deficit Hyperactivity Disorder (ADHD) at age 5. His parents are active members of a Fundamentalist church. Family life revolves around the church: Sunday services, Wednesday suppers, social events, and friends. Luke, who attends the church school, is impulsive, hyperactive, and easily distracted. He frequently is sent to the principal's office for discipline, which usually consists of his having to memorize Bible verses. His parents oppose giving him stimulant medication to treat his ADHD. His father believes strong discipline and prayer are the best ways to change a child's behavior. Luke's father used to whip him with a belt until someone reported him to the state's Child Protective Services. This agency forced Luke's father to get therapy and attend anger management and parenting classes in order to prevent Luke from being placed in a foster home.

About two years ago, Luke began to experience periodic bouts of eye blinking. No one in his family or at school paid attention to this behavior until a teacher noticed it and wondered if he needed eyeglasses. The school nurse checked his vision and found it to be normal, but she noticed Luke was clearing his throat a lot. The school nurse called this behavior to the attention of Luke's mother. The mother shared that she was worried about Luke because her uncle had Tourette's Disorder and she hoped her son did not have this same problem. She described her uncle as having no control over profanity and, when walking down the street, he would periodically spin around in the opposite direction, scratch his body, do some unusual jerks of the head, spin back around, and continue on his way. Luke's mother confessed she had noticed periodic eye blinking, head jerking, and barking like a dog well over a year ago, but had been reluctant to find out the cause. She hoped he did not begin cussing like his uncle, as Fundamentalist Baptists have very strict rules about cussing.

The school nurse suggests that Luke be seen by a child psychiatrist. The child psychiatrist diagnoses Luke with Tourette's Disorder. The psychiatrist suggests a yeast-free diet, a course of nystatin, and therapy with a mental health professional. Luke's father again says no to medication.

Case Study

Luke has not begun therapy with a mental health professional, instead he is starting a two-week church summer day camp. On the first day, he goes to see the camp nurse when he doesn't feel well. The camp nurse finds his vital signs are normal, but she hears Luke suddenly say a string of curse words. Minutes later, he barks like a dog. He tells the nurse, "I think I must be a bad dog in a boy's body." The nurse responds, "Hmmm, thank you for telling me what you are thinking about. Let me think about it a while.

In the meantime, how about shooting some baskets with me and maybe playing a game of horse in basketball?" Luke agrees to shoot some baskets. Later, the nurse reviews Luke's medical records and checks to see if he is on a yeast-free diet.

Questions

1. Why do you think the nurse suggested shooting baskets when Luke stated he thought he was a dog in a boy's body? What other responses would be appropriate? Why?

2. What is Luke's developmental stage according to Erickson? How would this information affect your response?

3. If you were the camp nurse, would you try to encourage a friendship with another camper? If so, would you encourage a male friendship over a female friendship? If so, why?

4. What does the word *tic* mean?

5. What are the diagnostic criteria for Tourette's Disorder (TD)?

6. How would you answer Luke's parents when they ask, "Are there more adults with TD than children? What is the usual course of TD? Does it affect boys more often than girls?"

7. Luke's parents ask you, "What causes TD? Is ADHD commonly associated with it? Can Luke be cured? What other conditions are commonly associated with TD?" How would you respond to these questions?

8. What treatments are currently being used with clients who have TD? What do you know about nystatin (Mycostatin) that might relate to treating TD?

9. What areas would you like to assess before writing a care plan for Luke? What nursing diagnoses would you likely write for him? What interventions would you include in a nursing care plan for Luke?

10. If you were the camp nurse, what teaching points would you like to communicate to Luke's parents in regard to his needs?

11. Luke's parents ask you to pray with them. How would you handle this request?

Questions and Suggested Answers

1. Why do you think the nurse suggested shooting baskets when Luke stated he thought he was a dog in a boy's body? What other responses would be appropriate? Why? The nurse suggested shooting baskets to distract Luke and to reduce his stress level. People with Tourette's Disorder (TD) tend to have fewer tics when they engage in activities. You could engage him in other activities besides basketball, such as working on a puzzle, playing cards, or caring for a camp pet. In addition to distracting and reducing stress, these activities present an opportunity to include another child later. Shooting baskets is especially good for a boy with ADHD, because he can burn some hyperactive energy and concentrate on a task.

You could respond to Luke's statement with an open-ended therapeutic communication tool (e.g., "Tell me more about this thought of being a bad dog in a boy's body). Luke's response could possibly help you learn the origin of this thought, such as something someone said to him. His statement could also be a clue to delusions or hallucinations, however, it is more likely that it reflects the thinking of a boy his age or a name he was called when making barking sounds. Deciding to shoot baskets rather than explore the meaning of Luke's statement does not mean you can't explore the statement later. Hours later or days later, you could remind Luke of his statement and ask him to tell you more about it.

It is important to plant the idea with Luke that he is a good boy, so you might say, "I have confidence that you are a good boy in a boy's body."

2. What is Luke's developmental stage according to Erickson? How would this information affect what you say or do with him? Luke is at the stage of industry versus inferiority. A child in this stage of development learns to have self-worth by attaining mastery of psychosocial, physiologic, and cognitive skills. Thus, you and the camp staff should plan activities that Luke can master. Shooting baskets and gaining skills in basketball is one kind of mastery. Learning a Bible verse or working on a project in pairs are other kinds of mastery. Learning how to talk with his parents and peers is another kind of mastery. You should give Luke encouraging feedback. You want to model the behavior you want to see in Luke. You can role-play with him about how he can get his parents' attention and talk with them, and how to communicate with a peer. If Luke misses a basket but tried hard, you could point out that you like his concentration or that it was a very good try.

3. If you were the camp nurse, would you try to encourage a friendship with another camper? If so, would you encourage a male friendship over a female friendship? If so, why? In the industry versus inferiority stage, children are becoming society and peer focused. A 10-year-old boy greatly benefits from having a best friend of the same gender. In Henry Stack Sullivan's stages of interpersonal theory of development, Luke is in preadolescence (9–12), a stage in which a child is vulnerable to teasing and when a "chum" is important (Potts and Mandelco, 2002).

4. What does the word *tic* mean? *Tics* are uncontrollable vocal sounds (also referred to as phonic) or involuntary motor movements. Motor tics usually begin in the face, but can later involve any part of the body. Simple motor tics include eye blinking, head jerking, and facial grimacing. Complex motor tics include squatting, twirling during walking, and deep knee bends. Vocal tics include yelps, snorts, coughs, barks, throat clearing, and hiccups. Medina (2004), who includes shrugs as tics, says that people with TD commonly experience obsessive thoughts. Bruun and associates (2005) include humming, palm licking, and poking or pinching the genitals as tics.

About 10 percent of people with TD have coprolalia, which is the explosive utterance of obscenities or racial slurs. This sign is not needed for a diagnosis of TD, although the person for whom the disorder is named, a French doctor George Gilles de la Tourette, had coprolalia. A person can have either vocal tics or motor tics (not both) and not be diagnosed with TD. The *Diagnostic and Statistical Manual of Mental Disorders* (APA, 2000) refers to the condition as Tourette's Disorder whereas professional and popular literature use Tourette's Syndrome.

5. What are the diagnostic criteria for TD? The criteria that must be met to receive a diagnosis of Tourette's Disorder are:

1. Have had multiple motor and at least one vocal tic, not necessarily both occurring concurrently but at some time during the illness.
2. Have experienced tics many times during the day almost every day or intermittently for more than twelve months, never free of the tics for more than three months in a row.
3. The tics must have begun prior to age 18.
4. The tics must not be due to substance use or a medical condition.

The diagnosis for just motor tics or just vocal tics, yet meeting criteria two through four above and never having met the criteria for TD, will be termed as Chronic Motor or Vocal Tic Disorder. There also is Transient Tic Disorder (TTD) in which the severity of the symptoms and the duration are less than in TD. TTD can last as little as four weeks but no longer than twelve consecutive months.

The more a child with TD attempts to control the behavior, the more evident the behavior is. Semon (2005, 2) explains the phenomenon by saying, "For a tic to occur, a center in the brain must fire, triggering the muscles to move. In normal individuals such centers do not fire involuntarily." This is because most of the brain is devoted to keeping the brain ready to work but not working. In TD, the inhibitory function of the brain is decreased, allowing the brain to fire and initiate a behavior that was not called for.

6. How would you answer Luke's parents when they ask, "Are there more adults with TD than children? What is the usual course of TD? Does it affect boys more often than girls?" More children than adults have TD, with the incidence being reported as five to thirty individuals per ten thousand children compared to one to two individuals per ten thousand adults (APA, 2000). Bruun and colleagues (2005) state that transient tic disorders can occur in up to 18 percent of children.

TD can commence as early as age 2, but it is usually found during childhood or early adolescence before age 18. Onset median age is approximately age 6 to 7. This disorder can last throughout the person's life, although periods of remission lasting weeks to years can occur (APA, 2000). In some cases, the symptoms disappear by early adulthood; in others, the symptoms lessen in severity, variety, disruptiveness, and frequency. The National Institute of Neurological Disorders and Stroke (NINDS; 2006) websites relates, "Although TS is generally lifelong and chronic, it is not degenerative. In a few cases, complete remission occurs after adolescence."

In clinical settings, TD is diagnosed about three to five times more frequently in males compared to females. In the community, it is on the order of two to one (APA, 2000).

7.　Luke's parents ask you, "What causes TD? Is ADHD commonly associated with it? Can Luke be cured? What other conditions are commonly associated with TD?" How would you respond to these questions? The exact cause of TD is unknown. It is generally thought to have a genetic connection. The National Institute of Neurological Disorders and Stroke states, "Tourette Syndrome is an inherited neurological disorder (NINDS, 2006). Leckman (2002) relates that speculation on cause has included toxic substances irritating motor neural systems, subcortical structure differences, and subcortical structure differences as well as heredity. Semon (2005) theorizes that yeast in the body slows the brain's neuronal firing down and this is the cause of the tics that will diminish or disappear with anti-yeast therapy.

Potts and Mandelco (2002) report that as many as 8 percent of autistic children have TD. Obsessive-Compulsive Disorder also is associated with TD, with some clients with TD having Obsessive-Compulsive Disorder concurrently.

There is no cure for TD, but it is possible to reduce the associated symptoms. Many clients with TD show improvement with treatment or with time. In some cases, TD goes into complete remission.

8.　What treatments are currently being used with clients who have TD? What do you know about nystatin that might relate to treating TD? Relaxation techniques and biofeedback are two of the least controversial treatments being used to reduce clients' signs and symptoms. According to NINDS (2006), most people with TD do not require medication, but narcoleptic drugs and antihypertensive drugs are used for clients whose symptoms interfere with their functioning. These drugs have long-term and short-term side effects, which practitioners, clients, and parents of minor children must weigh against the benefits. The newer narcoleptics seem to have fewer side effects than earlier narcoleptics such as haloperidol (Haldol), which once was the drug of choice for treating TD. Stimulants are used in some cases.

Semon (2005) describes treating several cases of TD successfully with nystatin, better food choices, and eliminating yeast products. Nystatin

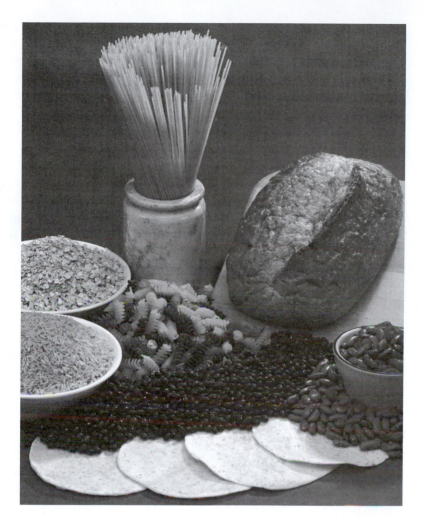

is given to adults with an overgrowth of yeast in the digestive system. Yeast, a normal component of the digestive system, can grow more rapidly after taking antibiotics or when a person eats a diet high in sugar or has diabetes. Regardless of whether anti-yeast treatments such as nystatin alleviate signs and symptoms of TD, all children, including children with TD and ADHD, need to limit their sugar intake.

9. What areas would you like to assess before writing a care plan for Luke? What nursing diagnoses would you likely write for him? What interventions would you include in a nursing care plan for Luke? You need to asses the family strengths, dynamics, beliefs, and limitations as well as Luke's talents and strengths; psychosocial, physical, and spiritual needs; and educational strengths and needs. You could assess his behaviors related to his stage of development and his beliefs in terms of stage of moral development.

Nursing diagnoses would include: Body Image Disturbed; Knowledge Deficit related to TD; Loneliness; Risk for Parenting Impaired; or Parenting readiness for enhanced.

The Nemours Foundation (2004) suggests five areas appropriate for intervention:

1. Involvement. Remember the camp nurse getting Luke involved in shooting baskets? Tics can be fewer and milder when the client's mental and physical energy is focused on sports or hobbies.
2. Helping others. Children with TD tend to be understanding of other people's feelings. Nurses and parents can encourage them to volunteer when appropriate.
3. Engagement in creative activities. Writing, playing a musical instrument, and painting can help focus the mind on things other than stressful events or tics.
4. Getting support. There is a Tourette's Syndrome Association.
5. Control. People with Tourette's can feel more in control if they learn more about TD, ask their health care provider lots of questions, and be active in their treatment. In this case, the parents as well as the client will benefit from education about TD and participating in treatment planning and intervention.

Additional interventions include helping the child develop strategies for explaining the tics to peers via role playing and scripted conversations.

10. If you were the camp nurse, what teaching points would you like to communicate to Luke's parents in regard to his needs? Helpful teaching points include:

- Nurturing, positive, consistent interactions with Luke are important.
- Calling attention to his tics and insisting that he control them will only make the tics worse. Scolding a child about tics also makes them worse.
- It is best to be sensitive and supportive of the child with tics.
- Tics are less frequent when the child relaxes; tics do not appear during sleep (Schor, 1999).
- Playing with your child is important. It helps you better understand your child, and it communicates to your child that he is important to you.
- Children learn through play. Age-appropriate games can help the child learn to concentrate, master new material, and organize his thoughts. Adult minds also benefit from games.

- All children, including Luke, need special friends with which to share ideas, wants, secrets, and experiences. Parents can be taught how to facilitate this interaction.

11. Luke's parents ask you to pray with them. How would you handle this request? There is no correct answer. In this situation, you are the church camp nurse so you probably feel comfortable praying. If you don't, you could ask the pastor or the youth leader of the church to pray with the family. In your own life and work, you may or may not feel comfortable praying with or for others. You need to discuss this with your instructor or a peer.

References

American Psychiatric Association (APA). (2000). *Diagnostic and Statistical Manual of Mental Disorders, 4th ed.* Text Revision. Washington, DC: American Psychiatric Association.

Bruun, R. D., et al. (2005). "Guide to the Diagnosis and Treatment of Tourette Syndrome." www.tsa-usa.org/research/guidetodiagnosis.html. Accessed June 16, 2006.

Leckman, J. F. (2002). "Tourette's Syndrome." *Lancet* 360(9345): 1577–1587.

Medina, J. (2004). "Molecules of the Mind: Profiling Tourette's Syndrome." *Psychiatric Times* 121:14, 40–41.

National Institute of Neurological Disorders and Stroke (NINDS). (2006). "NINDS Tourette Syndrome Information Page." www.ninds.nih.gov/disorders/tourette/tourette.htm. Accessed June 15, 2006. Nemours Foundation. (2004). "Tourette Syndrome." www.kidshealth.org/parent/medical/brain/tourette.html. Accessed January 21, 2005.

Potts, N. L. and B. L. Mandelco. (2002). *Pediatric Nursing: Caring for Children and Their Families.* Clifton Park, N.J: Thomson Delmar Learning.

Schor, E. L., ed. (1999). "Tics." In *Caring for Your School Age Child: Ages 5–12.* New York: Bantam. Available online at www.medem.com.

Semon, B. (2005). "Yeast and Tourette's Syndrome." www.nutritioninstitute.com/Tourettes_Syndrome.html. Accessed June 17, 2006.

CASE STUDY 3

William

MODERATE

GENDER

M

AGE

75

SETTING

- Retirement community

ETHNICITY

- Black American

CULTURAL CONSIDERATIONS

- Black American culture
- Church culture
- Military culture

PREEXISTING CONDITION

COEXISTING CONDITION

- Prostate cancer

COMMUNICATION

- Wears hearing aids

DISABILITY

SOCIOECONOMIC

- Upper middle class

SPIRITUAL/RELIGIOUS

- Was a church deacon for many years
- Stopped attending church since move to the retirement community

PHARMACOLOGIC

PSYCHOSOCIAL

- Loss of contact with family and friends since move to retirement community

LEGAL

- A nurse can be prosecuted for aiding in a suicide

ETHICAL

- Does a person have the right to commit suicide?

ALTERNATIVE THERAPY

PRIORITIZATION

DELEGATION

SPECIAL POPULATIONS: THE CHILD, ADOLESCENT, OR ELDERLY CLIENT

Level of difficulty: Moderate

Overview: Requires knowledge of the verbal, behavioral, and situational clues indicating a person is at risk of suicide, ability to assess the degree of risk, and skill in devising appropriate preventive interventions. The nurse must avoid control battles, build an alliance with the client, come up with a plan for checking on the safety of the client, and find a means of "anchoring" the client. Due to this client's hearing loss, the nurse also must develop ways to ensure the client understands what the nurse is communicating. If all preventive actions fail, the nurse must help staff and family work through feelings and process the suicide.

Client Profile

William is a 75-year-old male from the "Bible Belt." William faithfully attended both Sunday school and church every week as a child. After high school, he joined the military and stayed in the service for over twenty years. During that time he married and had two children. After his wife died, he lived alone. William became very lonely and decided to remarry at age 73. His new wife felt they were too old to cook and clean; she talked him into moving to a retirement community where they could live in a small apartment and take as many meals as they wished in the communal dinning hall.

William sold his home, his car, and most of his belongings. He even sold his gun collection, except for one favorite pistol. He hid it and some ammunition in his sock drawer. He told no one about the gun.

Shortly after moving to the retirement community, William decided he hated living in a small apartment. He did not like the people who ate in the dining room, insisting that he and his wife sit alone at a table. He also was unhappy with his second wife. In fact, there was little in his life that made him happy except for playing chess once a week. He began to stay in bed most of the day unless it was his day to play chess.

During a routine visit to his health care provider, William learned he had prostate cancer. William did not tell his wife the news; instead, he encouraged her to go visit one of her children.

Case History

The day-shift nurse at the retirement center health care unit receives the report detailing William's prostate cancer. While reading it, the nurse recalls some data indicating there is a high rate of suicide in elderly white males after receiving this diagnosis. She doesn't think William is at risk for suicide because he is black American; nevertheless, the nurse telephones William and says, "I need to stop by and talk with you about your health care provider's diagnosis of prostate cancer." William replies, "That won't be necessary. It's all been taken care of. You won't have to worry about me any longer."

The nurse goes to the facility kitchen to find out what William's favorite foods are. The dietitian reveals that William likes sugar-free orange gelatin with mandarin oranges. The nurse takes a bowl to William's door, where William reluctantly invites her inside. After talking about the weekly chess game, the nurse offers to answer any questions William might have about prostate cancer. She assesses William for suicidal ideation and intent as well as risk factors. The nurse asks William to help her come up with a way to determine each day if he is all right. William asks the nurse, "Why do you have to check on me to see if I am alright? If I decide to kill myself, I should have the right to do it. I have prostate cancer and I am going to die anyway."

Two days later, William calls the nurse to check in; he tells her everything is wonderful. His mood seems much brighter to the nurse. At noon the following day, the nurse has security meet her at the door to William's apartment. William has not checked in with her that day.

Questions

1. Why did the nurse get William's favorite food and knock on his door unannounced? Why didn't the nurse just leave him alone as he requested?

2. Why does the nurse want William's help in designing a system to ensure he is all right each day? What kind of system could be implemented?

3. In addition to having trouble hearing the phone or door bell ring, what other problems does William's hearing difficulty pose for the nurse in light of his possible depression and suicidality? What nursing interventions would be helpful?

4. How should you respond when William asserts his right to kill himself? What are the legal and ethical implications of ignoring suicidal clues or assisting a client in committing suicide? What actions should the nurse take if she determines the client is suicidal, has a plan, and intends to carry it out?

5. How would you respond to William's statement that he'll die anyway from prostate cancer? What is prostate cancer? Does it affect black Americans differently?

6. What clues indicate a person is suicidal? What are some risk factors for suicide? Does William exhibit any risk factors?

7. What role could culture play in this case?

8. If you were the nurse, what assessment data would you want to gather on this client?

9. What nursing diagnoses, goals, and interventions would you write for this client?

10. What emotions might be present in a nurse working with a suicidal client? What emotions might the nurse and family members experience if the client successfully commits suicide? What actions does the nurse need to take when a client commits suicide?

Questions and Suggested Answers

1. Why did the nurse get William's favorite food and knock on his door unannounced? Why didn't the nurse just leave him alone as he requested? The nurse wants to have a face-to-face talk with William. He has indicated he does not want to talk to the nurse, and the nurse doubts he will come to see her, so she must be invited inside William's apartment to assess his mental state and risk of suicide. Taking a favorite food is a way of throwing William off guard and getting herself invited inside. The food keeps the topic light and safe at first, hopefully keeping the client from becoming defensive as the nurse shifts into assessment. This approach allows the nurse to avoid a control battle with the client by telling him to expect a visit when he has insisted the nurse not make a visit.

William gave the nurse at least one clue that he could be suicidal when he said, "It's all been taken care of. You won't have to worry about me any longer." The nurse must take this clue seriously and assess the client quickly.

The nurse could have taken William a book on a favorite topic such as chess or bring him an article she wants to talk to him about.

2. Why does the nurse want William's help in designing a system to ensure he is all right each day? What kind of system could be implemented? The nurse needs a system to check on William each day because he is temporarily living alone, tends to isolate in his room, is hard of hearing, usually refuses to wear hearing aids, could be depressed, and might be thinking of hurting himself. The nurse wants William's input because this strategy will ensure greater client compliance with the system. Any system is acceptable. In one design, William could call the switchboard or the nurse each day. This approach is preferable to the nurse placing the call due to William's difficulty in hearing the phone. In some assisted-living facilities, a staff member places a card atop the client's door each night. The card will fall when the door is next opened. If the card has not fallen by an agreed-on time the next morning, a staff member will ring the doorbell. If there is no answer, security will come and unlock the door to check on the client.

3. In addition to having trouble hearing the phone or door bell ring, what other problems does William's hearing difficulty pose for the nurse in light of his possible depression and suicidality? What nursing interventions would be helpful? William's hearing difficulty could cause him to hear something totally different than what the nurse said. Thus, the nurse needs to ask William to repeat what she says to ensure he has processed the correct information. Making sure the message sent is the message received is important in any nurse–client communication, but it is especially important with the suicidal client.

The nurse can help the client hear better by facing him when talking and standing close to the ear with better hearing. The nurse can ask to see his hearing aids and check them to ensure they are working properly and the batteries are good. The nurse could then say, "I need you to turn on your hearing aids for a few minutes." Being directive without being "bossy" works better with suicidal and depressed clients than offering them a choice such as, "Would you like to turn your hearing aids on?" If you ask a question, you must be prepared for a negative response.

4. How should the nurse respond when William asserts his right to kill himself? What are the legal and ethical implications of ignoring suicidal clues or assisting a client in committing suicide? What actions should the nurse take if she determines the client is suicidal, has a plan, and intends to

carry it out? The law is clear: A nurse cannot legally assist a client in killing himself. In fact, the nurse can be named in a lawsuit for contributing to the death of a client who commits suicide if the nurse did not respond to the client's suicidal clues as a reasonable and prudent nurse would. Ethically, you as a nurse are charged with preserving life. It is not for you to decide if a person can take his own life or under what circumstances.

You could respond to this client's comment by saying, "So, have you thought about killing yourself?" You must stay silent and allow the client time to respond. Silence is an effective therapeutic communication tool for eliciting information. Another acceptable approach is to ask the client directly if he is thinking about killing himself, saying, "Are you thinking about killing yourself now?" If the response is negative, you might want to ask, "Have you ever thought about killing yourself recently or in the past?" If the client admits to being suicidal, you need to determine if the client has a plan and a method in mind. You could ask, "Do you have a method in mind? If so, what is it?" The client will either respond negatively or will actually tell you he is thinking about shooting himself. Your next questions should be, "Do you have a gun or have you thought about getting one? Do you have ammunition?" If William admits to having a plan to shoot himself and having a gun and ammunition, you then should ask, "Where do you keep this gun?" You have to consider the danger of asking William to surrender the gun to you. It could go off accidentally, or William could be homicidal as well as suicidal. It is time to problem solve quickly. One good option is to separate William from his gun. You could think of a way to get William out of the apartment and busy in activities in the facility. You then need to notify your supervisor, the administrator, and the client's health care provider. The facility might have a policy for dealing with this situation. Or, the health care provider could order a search of William's apartment.

Someone can tactfully explain this weapon confiscation to William later, letting him know that the weapon will be secured for him in a safe place. Then, the health care provider must assess William's suicide intent to determine if he needs to have a caregiver with him twenty-four hours a day, some interim means of checking on him, or be admitted to a psychiatric facility.

5. How would you respond to William's statement that he'll die anyway from prostate cancer? What is prostate cancer? Does it affect black Americans differently? You should respond by suggesting that the two of you form an alliance to get more information about prostate cancer and options for treatment. You also should suggest that you and he discuss treatment options with his health care provider to see which option he prefers and would be best for him. Methods of treatment include radical prostatectomy, external beam radiation, cryotherapy, seed implants, and chemotherapy.

You need to ask William, "When you think about prostate cancer, what do you imagine?" Then, he can talk freely about his fears. His response also will provide an idea of what he knows about this disease and what misconceptions he holds. You also need to ask about his symptoms. He could be asymptomatic or symptomatic (e.g., difficulty urinating, urinary frequency, difficulty starting or maintaining a stream of urine, in pain).

Selley and colleagues (1997) report that the worldwide incidence of prostate cancer rose in the late 1990s, likely because of the growing elderly population and an increased prostate specific antigen testing (PSA). National Human Genome Research Institute (2006) indicates that prostate cancer is the most common cancer in black American males, most often affecting men over age 65. In addition, there is a relatively unstudied form of early-onset familial prostate cancer that occurs in black Americans. Another report (Senior Journal, 2005) indicates that some types of cancer, including prostate cancer, are still rising even though the overall incidence of cancer is relatively stable.

Black American men have double the incidence of prostate cancer compared to white American males and twice the mortality rate. Healthy black American males tend not to receive prostate screening compared to white American males even when they have first-degree relatives with prostate cancer (Medical College of Georgia, 2006).

Research is being conducted into the possibility of a hereditary form of prostate cancer. Researchers at the National Human Genome Research Institute (2006) have located a gene called HPC-1, which, when altered, has been found to be associated with an increased risk of prostate cancer.

6. What clues indicate a person is suicidal? What are some risk factors for suicide? Does William exhibit any risk factors? Suicidal clues can be verbal, behavioral, or situational. Verbal clues include statements such as, "I don't have any friends anymore, and there is nothing good in my life anymore." or "You won't have to worry about me much longer." Behavioral clues include prior suicide attempts, hoarding pills or buying a gun, and an inability to visualize the future when asked to describe what life will be like six or twelve months from now. Other behavioral clues include giving away prized possessions, making a will or writing an obituary, and acting differently (e.g., more secretive, mood swings, or increased somatic complaints). Situational clues include a change of living location that is perceived as unhappy or bad, loss of a significant other, diagnosis of a chronic or terminal illness, and chronic pain.

Suicide rates are higher in males than females. Females are more likely to attempt suicide and males more likely to complete it. Having a first-degree relative who committed suicide is considered a risk factor. Black American and Native Indian males rank highest for suicide among adolescents and young adults. In the older adult, white males outnumber black Americans in completed suicides. Gibbs (1997) discusses suicide among black Americans and suggests there is a trend toward increased suicide in very elderly blacks, particularly males, as well as adolescents. At one time, the rate of black American suicides was one fourth that of white males, but it now stands at one half. In black Americans age 65 and older, 74 percent of all suicides involved firearms. Notably, firearms comprised the most common suicide method among black Americans regardless of age or gender (American Association of Suicidology, 2004).

Barnes and Bell (2003) discuss an unreplicated 1987 study by Rothberg and associates in which the suicide rate for black military men ages 45 to 55 was 4.5 times higher than that of white military men of the same age group. Perhaps being black American, elderly, male, and ex-military are risk factors for William.

William might be at risk for suicide due to depressed mood, which needs further assessment. If he is depressed, it could be situational depression due to the loss of his wife, loss of contact with his children, relocation, and/or his lack of happiness with his second marriage. Depression could be associated with receiving a diagnosis of cancer.

The National Institute of Mental Health (2003) states that depression is associated with suicide in the elderly, particularly when associated with chronic illness or side effects of medication. Depression is not a normal part of aging.

7. What role could culture play in this case? William was raised in a black American family in the South. Church and family are important. Southern living, family support, and spiritual connectivity are protective factors mitigating against suicide (Gibbs, 1997). William appears to have lost his connection to both church and family. He might have lost touch with the military and black cultures, too. Culture and cultural needs are important areas for assessment, as they hold implications for nursing interventions to anchor the client.

An *anchor* is something important to the client that keeps him focused on staying alive rather than wanting to kill himself. For example, having the client reestablish contact with family members, peers in the military, or a church similar to the one in which he grew up might give William something to live for. Simply talking to the nurse, staff, and others about the various cultures that he identifies with might be helpful. The nurse can help provide these discussion opportunities.

8. If you were the nurse, what assessment data would you want to gather on this client? You need to gather data on suicide risk on an ongoing basis, key aspects of which have been discussed above. You need to determine if there is any family history of suicide and depression and assess for depression. A spiritual needs assessment would be helpful. You need to gather data on any symptoms of prostate cancer that the client might be experiencing. The client's relationship with his current wife, as well as his relationship with the rest of his family, needs to be explored as well.

9.   What nursing diagnoses, goals, and interventions would you likely write for this client? Possible nursing diagnoses for this client include: Risk for Suicide; Ineffective Individual Coping; Risk for Powerlessness; Risk for Loneliness; Hopelessness; Fear; Relocation Stress Syndrome; Depressed Mood; Deficient Knowledge or Readiness for Enhanced Knowledge; and Spiritual Distress.

Goals for this client could include:

- Will not harm himself or others.
- Will reduce time isolating in room by participating in one outside activity per day.
- Will eat at least one meal per day in the common dining room.
- Will sit with at least one other person than his wife.
- Will discuss treatment options for prostate cancer with health care provider.
- Will make at least two contacts a week with family members.
- Will outline a plan to meet spiritual needs.

Interventions could include those already discussed in regard to (1) improving the client's chances of hearing the nurse and others accurately and (2) keeping the client safe (i.e., from committing suicide or harming himself or others in any way). An early intervention would be for the nurse to build a trusting relationship with the client, form an alliance to gather information about prostate cancer, and determine the best treatment for the client. Other interventions would include measures to reduce isolation and lift the client's mood (e.g., keeping the client informed in writing about facility activities such as field trips and encouraging him to sign up for activities of interest). People with depression often do better with quiet activities with one or two people rather than gregarious activities with a group. A nursing effort could be made to gradually introduce the client to other residents in the facility. Pet therapy might be helpful in lifting this client's mood. The health care provider can be consulted about the possibility of scheduled visits by a psychiatric nurse clinician or other mental health professional to do individual therapy and couples therapy with the client and his wife. The health care provider might order an antidepressant; if so, the nurse would provide education about the medication and ensure the client does not "cheek" the medication for use in an alternative suicide plan.

10. What emotions might be present in a nurse working with a suicidal client? What emotions might the nurse and family members experience if the client successfully commits suicide? What actions does the nurse need to take when a client commits suicide? The nurse might feel a wide range of emotions in working with a suicidal client. The nurse might fear that the client will commit suicide or feel empathy with the client. The nurse could be angry that the client would even consider this act, which once completed cannot be undone.

A common feeling is guilt. Family members question themselves about whether they could have done something to prevent the suicide; they also experience sadness, loss, and anger. The nurse can help herself and others resolve guilt and other feelings by scheduling a staff meeting to process the suicide as well as peoples' feelings and to learn how the staff might make changes to better prevent suicides in the future. Notification of the client's death, including the factual circumstances of the death, must be made.

References

American Association of Suicidology. (2004). "African American Suicide Fact Sheet." www.suicidology.org/associations/1045/files/AfricanAmer2002.pdf. Accessed February 9, 2006.

Barnes, D. H. and C. C. Bell. (January 2003). "Paradoxes of Black Suicide." *Preventing Suicide—The National Journal.* 1/1/03.

Gibbs, J. T. (1997). "African-American Suicide: A Cultural Paradox." *Suicide and Life-Threatening Behavior* 27(1): 68–79.

Medical College of Georgia. (2006). "High-Risk Black Men Are Screened Less for Prostate Cancer." www.eurekalert.org/pub_releases/2006-02/mcog-hbm020306.php. Accessed June 17, 2006.

National Human Genome Research Institute. (2006). "National Cooperative Study of Hereditary Prostate Cancer in African-Americans." www.genome.gov/10002040. Accessed February 21, 2006.

National Institute of Mental Health. (2003) "Older Adults: Depression and Suicide Facts." www.nimh.nih.gov/publicat/elderlydepsuicide.cfm. Accessed February 9, 2006.

Selley, S., et al. (1997). "Diagnosis, Management, and Screening of Early Localized Prostate Cancer." *Health Technology Assessment* 1(2): 1–96.

Senior Journal. (2005). "Cancer Trends 2005: New Cancer Report Sees Declining Deaths, Stable Incidence Rates". www.seniorjournal.com/NEWS/Health/5-12-23-CancerReport2005.htm. Accessed June 17, 2006.

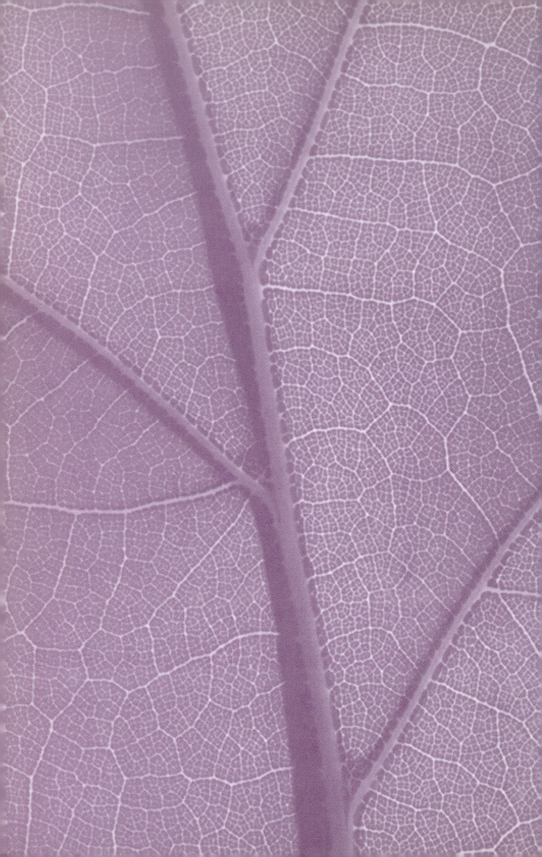

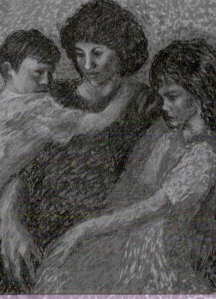

PART NINE

Survivors

of Violence

or Abuse

CASE STUDY 1

Janine

GENDER

F

AGE

23

SETTING

- Inpatient medical unit

ETHNICITY

- White American

CULTURAL CONSIDERATIONS

PREEXISTING CONDITION

- Diabetes Mellitus

COEXISTING CONDITION

- Diabetes Mellitus

COMMUNICATION

DISABILITY

SOCIOECONOMIC

- Middle class
- Working and going to graduate school

SPIRITUAL/RELIGIOUS

- Parents belong to Scientology church
- Client rejected Scientology in adolescence

PHARMACOLOGIC

- Zolpidem (Ambien)
- Levonorgestrel (Plan B)

PSYCHOSOCIAL

- Is outgoing and social
- Eats and drinks alcohol with friends; Diabetes gets out of control
- Drinking increases risk for rape

LEGAL

- Client: Decision of whether or not to bring charges against perpetrator
- Nurse: Charting and testimony might be used in court
- Confidentiality: Client has asked nurse not to reveal that she has been raped

ETHICAL

- Emergency contraception for rape
- Abortion
- Influencing client's decision versus providing information

ALTERNATIVE THERAPY

PRIORITIZATION

DELEGATION

MODERATE

SURVIVORS OF VIOLENCE OR ABUSE

Level of difficulty: Moderate

Overview: Requires the ability to be professional, objective, and adhere to legal and hospital protocols, yet be empathic and therapeutic with a client who describes being raped. Requires the ability to keep an open mind and use the nursing process to find out what is going on with the client instead of accepting others' negative view of the client.

225

Client Profile

Janine is a 23-year-old graduate student with Diabetes Mellitus. She has been admitted to the hospital several times in the past when her Diabetes was out of control. Janine has shared with several nurses that she eats foods that are not on her diet, goes to parties where she drinks beer, and corrects for these behaviors by giving herself extra units of regular insulin. She admits that sometimes she forgets to take her insulin and that she has not managed her diabetes very well.

Two days ago, two popular football players sexually abused Janine. They gave her a ride home from a fraternity party and raped her when they arrived at her apartment. She did not report the rape. Instead, she went to work and school the next day. She tried to forget the rape by pushing it to the back of her mind and keeping herself busy.

Janine holds a responsible position in an insurance company and goes to graduate school part time to earn a master's degree in business. She is nearing graduation. Recently, she met a boy that she likes and began thinking about marriage and children. Before the rape, she was thinking about managing her Diabetes better so she could have children.

Janine's parents belong to the Church of Scientology. Janine rejected the church when she was an adolescent.

Case Study

At 11 PM during the change of shift report, the 3–11 nurse tells the night nurse coming on duty that Janine, one of her assigned clients, is very attention seeking and noncompliant with her treatment regimen. About two hours into the shift, the night nurse hears Janine screaming. When the night nurse enters the room, Janine says she has had a bad dream and does not think she can get back to sleep. She says she is very anxious. She has a sleeping pill ordered (zolpidem 10 mg), which may be repeated one time for insomnia. She has not had a sleeping pill tonight.

Questions

1. How should you respond to a report that a client is attention seeking and non-compliant?

2. Should you give her zolpidem and go on break or do something else? What do you need to know about zolpidem?

3. You ask the client if there is anything bothering her that might have caused the nightmare. The client replies, "You wouldn't understand. You haven't experienced what I have." What do you say or do? Later, the client says, "I am going to tell you something that I haven't told anyone. I want you to promise not to tell anyone else." How should you respond?

Questions (continued)

4. The client reveals to you that two men raped her about forty-eight hours ago and she did not report it to the police. What do you say or do, if anything? Does this client have the right not to report being raped? What ethical issues are involved that might be troubling you or the client?

5. You recall there is a morning after pill (levonorgestrel) to prevent unwanted pregnancy. How long after sexual intercourse is this pill effective? Does this pill present any ethical or legal issues for you, the client, other nurses, the physician, the pharmacist, and/or the hospital?

6. What factors or variables increase an adult's vulnerability to sexual abuse? What are date rape drugs, and what educational tips could you give this client on preventive measures to avoid being given a date rape drug?

7. How common is sexual assault of an adult in the United States? How common is it for a victim of a sexual assault not to report the abuse to law enforcement? Why don't victims want to report an assault?

8. The client talks to you about her resolve to manage her Diabetes better. She says she is thinking about marrying her boyfriend and getting her sugar in good control so she can have a baby. What do you say or do?

9. What assessment data would you like on this client?

10. What nursing diagnoses would you write for this client? What goals would you write for this client?

11. What interventions do you think would be helpful in resolving likely nursing diagnoses and helping the client meet goals?

Questions and Suggested Answers

1. How should you respond to a report that a client is attention seeking and noncompliant? You need to keep an open mind and do your own assessment. Part of you might want to accept the information as true, but this information is subjective. It is human to have some negative thoughts about a client or a client's behavior as long as you don't act on them. Even if the client turns out to have observable behaviors suggestive of seeking attention or being noncompliant, you must remember that all behavior has meaning and purpose for the individual. You must find out what is behind this particular client's behavior.

When giving report at the end of your shift, you can model a professional manner of reporting that focuses on objective information, not how good the client is to the staff (sweet, pleasant, wonderful) or bad (demanding, uncooperative, complaining).

2. Should you give her zolpidem and go on break or do something else? What do you need to know about zolpidem? You need to help the client feel safe, and medication alone cannot do this. In this situation, it would be reassuring to the client if you stayed, pulled up a chair, and listened to the client. You could encourage the client to talk about the bad dream by using a therapeutic communication technique such as, "Tell me about your dream" or, "Tell me what is bothering you the most."

If you must go on break, you could ask the nurse relieving you to talk to the client while you are gone. However, the chances of the relief nurse talking to your client are not 100 percent, as she is responsible for many more clients while you are gone.

Zolpidem is a rapid-acting hypnotic sedative taken with a full glass of water. The client must lie down after taking it, and the bed's side rails need to be raised. This medication should not be taken on a full stomach, as this will delay its effect. If taken more than seven to ten days, this drug can be habit forming.

3. You ask the client if there is anything bothering her that might have caused the nightmare. The client replies, "You wouldn't understand. You haven't experienced what I have." What do you say or do? Later, the client says, "I am going to tell you something that I haven't told anyone else. I want you to promise not to tell anyone." How should you respond? It is not uncommon for people who have been raped to believe that no one can help them unless they've experienced rape. This is not true. You can say something like, "Perhaps I haven't experienced what you have. None of us have exactly the same experiences. I can listen closely to understand what you are going through and try to help you. Please talk with me and help me understand how I can help you."

You must tell the client that you cannot promise complete confidentiality. You must advise her that many things can be held in confidence, but if it affects her care or safety you must share this information with the client's health care provider, your supervisor, and possibly the health care team.

4. The client reveals to you that two men raped her about forty-eight hours ago and she did not report it to the police. What do you say or do, if anything? Does this client have the right not to report being raped? What ethical issues are involved that might be troubling you or the client? Even though the client has not reported this sexual abuse (rape) to the authorities, there can be future ethical and/or legal implications if you say or do nothing. The client could become pregnant, develop a sexually transmitted disease, or post traumatic stress disorder (PTSD), or could decide later to report the incident to legal authorities and press charges against the perpetrators. You need to share the information about the alleged rape with your supervisor immediately and with the health care provider. Hospital policy and your supervisor will be helpful in determining: (1) whether to wake the health care provider or wait until morning; and (2) what to chart.

Because the client is of legal age and mentally competent, she has the right not to report this rape. This is an ethical issue. These young men could rape other women in the future if they are not reported and convicted. You might feel strongly about pointing this possibility out to the client and asking her a lot of questions to find out why she is not going to report her rape. You should discuss these thoughts with your supervisor rather than acting on them. In the middle of the night, you need to listen to the client and reassure her that she is safe now. The issue can be explored later with the health care provider and/or primary nurse.

Another troubling and related issue is the possibility of sexually transmitted disease and the need to test perpetrators of rape for sexually transmitted disease. Diaz and associates (2004) point out yet another issue, which can pose ethical dilemmas for nurses: sexually victimized adolescents often do not tell their health care providers about sexual abuse. As a result, they do not get the medical treatment and psychological counseling that they need. This also is true of young adult and middle-aged women.

5. You recall there is a morning after pill (levonorgestrel) to prevent unwanted pregnancy. How long after sexual intercourse is this pill effective? Does this pill present any ethical or legal issues for you, the client, other nurses, the physician, the pharmacist, and/or the hospital? Levonorgestrel (Plan B) prevents unwanted pregnancy if taken within seventy-two hours of unprotected sexual intercourse. This medication stops ovulation and blocks implantation of any ovum already present. It is not effective once implantation has occurred. Two tablets are dispensed. One tablet is given as soon as possible within seventy-two hours of intercourse; the second tablet is given twelve hours later.

This client says she was raped two days ago. You need to find out exactly what time the rape occurred to know if emergency contraception is still an option. This information would affect your decision to call the health care provider right away or wait until morning.

This medication can present issues for professionals involved, as well as for the client. Some nurses feel strongly on both sides of the issue. Some religiously affiliated hospitals refuse to permit any form of abortion including a morning after pill. Some pharmacists refuse to dispense morning after pills based on personal beliefs that abortion is wrong. A 2004 case involved three Texas pharmacists who refused to honor a prescription for levonorgestrel based on moral and religious objections. At least four states—Georgia, Arkansas, South Dakota, and Mississippi—permit pharmacists to refuse to fill a prescription on the basis of personal beliefs. In contrast with United States practices, this drug is available over-the-counter in thirty-four countries (Zwillich, 2005).

If emergency contraception is an option and it is offered to this client, she might refuse to accept it based on religious beliefs or personal reasons. Some nurses will agree with this decision while others will not. They should talk to their supervisor or a professional counselor.

6. What factors or variables increase an adult's vulnerability to sexual abuse? What are date rape drugs, and what educational tips could you give this client on preventive measures to avoid being given a date rape drug? Higher rates of sexual victimization occur in adolescents who have sexual intercourse earlier with a number of sexual partners; who have mental, physical, or emotional disabilities; or who use alcohol or drugs (Raghavan et al., 2004). Arias (2004, 468) states, "Childhood maltreatment is a critical risk factor for physical and sexual victimization in adulthood."

Sawyer and colleagues (2002, 19) found that "although perpetrators of date rape can come from any part of the college community, two campus populations have been identified as possibly being high risk with regard to perpetrating sexual violence—fraternity members and athletes." However, these researchers also found that athletes were not homogeneous in their acceptance of rape myths. Athletes who play team sports are more likely to have ideas about sexual behaviors that make others more vulnerable to rape.

There are three major date rape drugs: flunitrazepam (Rohypnol), also known as Roofies, Ruffies, and R2; Gamma Hydroxy Butyrate (GHB), also called liquid Ecstasy, Liquid X, and X-rater; and ketamine hydrochloride, known as Ket, "K", and other street names. These drugs can be offered or slipped into drinks to enhance sexual desire and lessen the chances the victim will remember what happened. Other drugs, used in combination with alcohol, help lessen inhibitions and impair judgment, which can increase the chances of becoming a victim.

The nurse should recommend the following tips (McKinley Health Center, 2001) to clients:

1. Avoid mixed drinks and punch. They can have a high alcohol content and be laced with date rape or other drugs.
2. If you drink alcohol, select a drink of known alcohol content, know your limit, and limit yourself.
3. Select a trusted individual to be the designated driver who will not drink.
4. Do not accept a drink from an unknown person.
5. If someone around you is kidding about date rape drugs, pay attention and take this as a serious warning to get away from this person and this party.
6. Assess the behavior of others at a party. If they seem more intoxicated than the amount of drinking going on, this is a clue to leave.

7. How common is sexual assault of an adult in the United States? How common is it for a victim of a sexual assault not to report the abuse to law enforcement? Why don't victims want to report an assault? A recent article (*MMWR*, 2005, 311) states, "Rape is one of the most under reported crimes, making it difficult to accurately count the number of cases." The literature (Abby et al., 2005) also points out that:

- Sexual assault is very common in the United States.
- Most sexual assaults occur between people who know each other.
- Sexual assaults are usually not reported to the police.
- When sexual assaults are reported to the police very few perpetrators are incarcerated.

Kelly and associates (2005) cite a National Institute of Justice study that found 17.6 percent of females had experienced completed or attempted rape during their lifetime. In their own study of Navy personnel, they found that between 9.9 percent and 11.6 percent of male Navy recruits had raped a female prior to entering the military, which is about twice the rate for college men in general. In terms of attempted rape, the percentage was about 3.5 percent for both Navy recruits and college men. Some 53.1 percent of female Navy trainees reported being sexually victimized prior to age 17. Prior sexual victimization makes a woman more vulnerable to future rape.

One study of rape victims found that 84 percent did not report their rapes to the police. The main reason given was that "cultural norms . . . stigmatize and blame women for their assaults" (*MMWR*, 2005, 311). Women fear not being believed; and some have such low self-esteem and lack of knowledge about rape that they blame themselves and feel ashamed. Diaz and associates (2004, 171) found that it was "often necessary to correct the belief held by many victims that they were the only ones with these experiences and that they were somehow to blame." Other women fear that the perpetrator will get off free while they will pay the price of having their personal life made public and being traumatized by the police, and the court system.

While you can guess what possible thoughts the client is experiencing, you won't know until the client tells you. You should not jump to conclusions.

8. The client talks to you about her resolve to manage her Diabetes better. She says she is thinking about marrying her boyfriend and getting her sugar in good control so she can have a baby. What do you say or do? In regard to the client's motivation to comply with treatment, it should be encouraged. However, marriage and having a baby is a big step, especially for someone who has just been raped. The psychological and physical trauma of rape can affect the relationship with her boyfriend. You should encourage the client to seek couples counseling or premarital counseling as well as individual counseling.

9. What assessment data would you like on this client? The health care provider will either get an abuse history from the client or have the nurse elicit an abuse history. The rape might not be the first sexual abuse this client has experienced.

You need to explore what the client is feeling. Common feelings include anger and depression as well as helplessness, powerlessness, fear, and guilt. Still others feel dirty or violated. You should assess the client's body image and self-esteem. You also should assess the client's relationship with significant others. Zweig and colleagues (1999) stress the need to assess social/relational adjustment and feelings of anger, hostility, and depression in victimized women.

Identifying the client's strengths and limitations will be useful in helping her deal with the rape, manage Diabetes, and interact with others. You will want to look at the client's usual coping mechanisms and if they would be helpful now. In particular, the client's experience with managing Diabetes will be very helpful information. Her experience with rape could impact the degree of interest she has in complying with her treatment regimen. Yet, how she manages her Diabetes will impact her mood and the amount of energy she will have to deal with the rape experience.

10. What nursing diagnoses would you write for this client? What goals would you write for this client? Nursing diagnoses are based on assessment findings. However, common nursing diagnoses found in women who have been sexually assaulted include: Anxiety; Depression; Disturbed body image; Decisional conflict; Ineffective coping or Defensive coping; Ineffective denial; Fear; Ineffective health maintenance; Risk for infection; Readiness for enhanced knowledge; Risk for Rape-Trauma Syndrome (Compound or Silent Reaction); Readiness for enhanced religiosity; Situational low self-esteem; Disturbed sleep pattern; and Risk for sexual dysfunction. This client would be diagnosed with Ineffective Health Maintenance, as evidenced by her Diabetes being out of control, Ineffective Coping, Risk for Infection, and Disturbed Sleep Pattern. The Readiness for Enhanced Knowledge diagnosis also seems warranted.

Goals for this client could include:

- Will maintain Diabetes under control.
- Will discuss the rape with at least one trusted health professional and develop a plan for ongoing counseling.
- Will sleep six to eight hours each night without nightmares.
- Will adhere to treatment regimen for Diabetes.
- Will describe satisfaction with her body when she looks into a mirror or at least show progress in feeling more satisfied.
- Will be able to give at least two positive affirmations when asked to do so.

- Will be free of signs and symptoms of infection.
- Will identify two acceptable therapeutic means of dealing with feelings such as anger, depressions, fear, etc.

11. What interventions do you think would be helpful in resolving likely nursing diagnoses and helping the client meet goals? The following interventions could prove helpful:

- Build a trusting relationship with client and significant others.
- Focus on coming across as nonjudgmental.
- Model problem solving, and teach client problem solving.
- Encourage sharing of feelings by modeling and positive feedback
- Help client work through concerns about possible sexually transmitted disease and to get information regarding options for testing and prevention.
- Avoid revictimizing client with critical statements.
- Focus on helping client be and feel safe.
- Advocate for client.
- Help client learn to make positive affirmations to build self-esteem.
- Encourage client to identify and use talents.
- Teach client how to reduce vulnerability to sexual assaults through
  – Sexual Abuse Survivor Group
  – Assertiveness Training Group
  – Women's Issues Group
- Teach about sleeping medication.
- Encourage client to explore relationship with boyfriend through couple's therapy.
- Encourage client to explore spiritual needs and how to meet these needs.
- Put yourself in client's place and try to understand client's needs and behavior.

References

Abby, A., et al. (2005). "The Effects of Past Sexual Assault Perpetration and Alcohol Consumption on Men's Reactions to Women's Mixed Signals." *Journal of Social and Clinical Psychology* 24(2): 129–155.

Arias, I. (2004). "The Legacy of Child Maltreatment: Long-Term Health Consequences for Women." *Journal of Women's Health* 13(50): 468–473.

Diaz, A., et al. (2004). "Obtaining a History of Sexual Victimization from Adolescent Females Seeking Routine Health Care." *Mt Sinai J Medicine* 71(3): 170–173.

Kelly, M. L., et al. (2005). "An Evaluation of a Sexual Assault Prevention and Advocacy Program for U.S. Navy Personnel." *Military Medicine* 170(4): 320–327.

McKinley Health Center. (2001). "Date Rape Drugs—What You Need to Know About Them." http://www.mckinley.uiuc.edu/Handouts/date_rape_drugs.html. Accessed June 10, 2005.

"Notice to Readers: Sexual Assault Awareness Month—April 2005." (2005). *Morbidity and Mortality Weekly Report* 54(12): 311.

Raghavan, R., et al. (2004). "Sexual Victimization Among a National Probability Sample of Adolescent Women." *Perspectives on Sexual and Reproductive Health* 36(6): 225–231.

Sawyer, R. G., et al. (2002). "Rape Myth Acceptance Among Intercollegiate Student Athletes: A Preliminary Examination." *American Journal of Health Studies* 18(1): 19–26.

Zweig, J. M., et al. (1999). "A Longitudinal Examination of the Consequences of Sexual Victimization for Rural Young Adult Women." *Journal of Sex Research* 36(4): 396–399.

Zwillich, T. (2005). "U.S. Pharmacies Vow to Withhold Emergency Contraception." *Lancet* 365(9472): 1677–1678.

Index